National and International Drug Safety Guidelines

1988 Edition

Susan Alder and Gerhard Zbinden

Institute of Toxicology

Swiss Federal Institute of Technology (ETH) and University of Zurich

CH-8603 Schwerzenbach, Switzerland

M.T.C. Verlag Zollikon 1988

G. Zbinden, Lenzenwiesstrasse 6, CH-8702 Zollikon, Switzerland

Acknowledgments

We are greatly indebted to many governmental officials, colleagues and friends who have provided us with regulatory guidelines and additional information on drug safety testing and registration requirements in their countries. Some have even provided English translations of documents that we could neither read nor understand. Particularly helpful information was received from:

Dr. J.T. Ahokas, Melbourne/Australia; Dr. E.J. Al-Kaliffa, Kuwait/Arabian Gulf; Prof. R. Bass, Berlin/FRG; Biomedizinische Forschungsgesellschaft, Linz/Austria; Dr. J. Borvendeg, Budapest/Hungary; Prof. A. Canysz, Warsaw/Poland; Mr. H. Davis, Rockville/USA; Dr G Deltour, Evreux/France; Ms M.C. Donnelly, Brussels/Belgium; Dr. R.A. Drost, Rijkswijk/The Netherlands; Dr. N. Dusitsin, Bangkok/Thailand; Dr. F. Endrünyi, Budapest/Hungary; Prof. H. Frohberg, Darmstadt/FRG; Mr. D. Galletis, Zimbabwe/Africa; Ms. J. Genoud-Hames, Luxembourg/Luxembourg; Dr. V.C. Glocklin, Rockville/USA; Mr. P. Grech, Paris/France; Mr. R.C. Griffith, Wellington/New Zealand; Dr. S. Guo-Wei, Zhejiang/China; Dr. P.K. Gupta, New Delhi/India; Dr. M.R. Hamid, Cairo/Egypt; Dr. Y. Harada, Osaka/Japan; Mr. P. Hlavats, Ottawa/Canada; Mr. J. Hohnert, Konstanz/FRG; Mr. K. Holttinen, Helsinki/Finland; Dr. K. Jayasena, Peradeniya/Sri Lanka; Dr. D.B. Jefferys, London/UK; Dr. Pu-Young Kim, Seoul/Korea; Mr. E. Kkalos, Nicosia/Cyprus; Mrs. J. St. Kraus, Rockville/USA; Dr. Y.S. Kuan, Cuppage Center/Singapore; Mr. K.Y. Li, Hong Kong; Dr. M.G. Lie Hon Fong, Paramaribo/Suriname; Dr. E. Lindgren, Stockholm/Sweden; Dr. I. Lobato, Madrid/Spain; Mr. R.M. Mohabir, Port-of-Spain/Trinidad; Prof. C. Munoz, Santiago/Chile; Ms. L. Mylne, Oslo/Norway; Mr. D.F. Natabou, Cotonou/Benin; Dr. A. Nava, Nerviano/Italy; Mr. R. Oktem, Bakanliklar-Ankara/Turkey; Mr. I.J. Petersen, Reykjavik/Iceland; Dr. V. Ramirez, San Jose/Costa Rica; Prof. J. Richter, Berlin/GDR; Prof. M. Roberfroid, Brussels/Belgium; Ms. C.C. Sanchez, Manila/Philippines; Mr. T. Sangthongtong, Bangkok/Thailand; Dr. J.S. Sobrino, Madrid/ Spain; Dr. L. Szekeres, Szeged/Hungary; Dr. Schorn, Bonn/FRG; Prof. J.S. Schou, Copenhagen/Denmark; Drs. M. and S. Tannhauser, Porto Alegre/Brasil; Dr. O. Westbye, Oslo/Norway; Dr. Yee Shen Kuan, Cuppage Center/Singapore; Ms. J. Yotaki, Athens/Greece; Director Geral, Ministry of Health, Lisboa/Portugal.

We thank them all for their help.

Grateful acknowledgment is made for permission from William Morrow & Company Inc., New York, to reprint an excerpt from Robert M. Pirsig's book «Zen and the Art of Motorcycle Maintenance. An Inquiry into Values», © 1974 by Robert M. Pirsig.

We thank Mr. Francis Beckett for editing the English text.

Copyright © by M.T.C. Verlag, G. Zbinden, Lenzenwiesstrasse 6, CH-8702 Zollikon, Switzerland. All rights reserved. Neither this work nor any part may be reproduced or transmitted in any form or by any means, electronic or mechanical, including microfilming or recording, or by any information storage and retrieval system without permission in writing from the publisher.
ISBN 3-907 03702 2.

Table of Contents

Preface	5
A Look Behind Drug Regulatory Guidelines	7
International Guidelines:	
European Economic Community, EEC	20
Nordic Guidelines (Denmark, Finland, Iceland, Norway, and Sweden)	33
National Guidelines:	
Australia	38
Austria	45
Belgium	48
Benin, People's Republic of	49
Brasil	50
Canada	52
Chile	66
China, People's Republic of	67
Costa Rica	76
Cyprus, Republic of	78
Denmark	79
Egypt	80
Federal Republic of Germany, FRG	81
Finland	84
France	85
German Democratic Republic, GDR	88
Great Britain, see U.K.	
Greece	89
Hong Kong	90
Hungary	91
Iceland	93
India	94
Italy	98
Japan	101
Kuwait	116
Luxembourg	118
Malaysia	119
Netherlands, the	124
New Zealand	125
Norway	127
Philippines, Republic of the	128
Poland	129
Portugal	131
Singapore	132
South Korea, Republic of	133
Spain	143
Sri Lanka	144
Suriname	146

Sweden	147
Switzerland	148
Taiwan	150
Thailand	151
Trinidad	152
Turkey	155
United Kingdom, UK	157
United States of America, USA	164
Zimbabwe	182
Toxicological Requirements of Biotechnology Products	183
Steroidal Contraceptive Drugs	188
Notification and Approval Procedures for Clinical Trials	190
Index	199

Preface

Industrial toxicology has two very different faces: first, it considers the new chemical's potential hazards for chemists and biologists and all others who work with it. At this stage, a preliminary assessment of the toxicological characteristics is made, and these are related to the projected future use of the compound. In some pharmaceutical companies, this has been developed into a well structured analysis of important adverse properties, an approach known as «toxicological screening», which complements the new drug selection process, hitherto mainly carried out by pharmacologists and medicinal chemists.

Once a new drug candidate has been targeted for clinical trials, the second and much more extensive task of the toxicologist begins; the compound now undergoes a series of toxicological tests that must provide evidence of safety in its intended use, and, at the same time, will lead to a voluminous «dossier» for submission to drug regulatory agencies. These studies, in contrast to those conducted in the early phase, must follow rigid rules that determine the design of the protocols and the quality standards of all aspects of the experimental work, including record keeping («good laboratory practice»).

The protocols employed for routine toxicological studies are based on time honored traditions and knowledge gained from experience with drugs already in clinical use. In addition, they follow the more or less explicit directions issued by national and international regulatory agencies. In this book, we present summaries of all the regulatory guidelines that we have been able to obtain over the last few years. This collection process was not easy, and had it not been for the help of many colleagues and friends, the incompleteness of this endeavour would be even more glaring. Our heartfelt thanks go to all those who have provided us with official documents and additional information.

National and international drug safety guidelines differ in many respects. Some give the bare minimum, indicating only general concepts of drug testing. Others include many technical details, and some even attempt to justify certain requirements by referring to scientific findings. The nomenclature used also varies significantly from country to country. In our summaries, we have attempted to introduce a certain degree of uniformity, but left, whenever possible, typical peculiarities of style, particularly in those cases where the exact meaning was not entirely clear. The summaries in this book reflect our best understanding of the message contained in the national and international guidelines. However, all those who wish to prepare a registration dossier for a specific regulatory agency are advised to consult the original documents.

We are also not sure that all summaries included in this book reflect the latest thinking of any given regulatory agency. Although we have made diligent efforts to verify the validity of the documents reviewed, we can give no guarantee that all our summaries are complete and up-to-date. As a matter of fact, we were informed by several agencies that their guidelines are presently under revision. We must, therefore, apologize for all errors and omissions contained in this book. At the same time, we ask all those with newer and more accurate information to share it with us. We would particularly like to hear from countries whose drug safety guidelines we were unable to obtain.

Many may ask why we, as members of an academic institution, have spent so much time in order to collect and publish official drug safety guidelines that have little if anything to do with the research we conduct. One of the reasons is our obligation to train future industrial toxicologists. While we would prefer to teach only the fascinating scientific aspects of toxicology, we cannot spare them the hard realities of industrial drug safety testing. Thus, we must be fully informed of the requirements of governmental agencies.

A second and much more important reason is our conviction that drug safety testing as it is conducted now, and as it is regulated in national and international guidelines, is in great need of a thorough overhaul. This process has begun with a revision of requirements and protocols of acute toxicity testing. We are happy that the results of this activity are already clearly reflected in several safety guidelines. There are many other shortcomings in the current practice of industrial toxicology. It is our goal to track them down in official documents, to put them up for discussion, and to encourage research into better procedures. We sincerely hope that some of our readers will join us in this adventure.

Schwerzenbach, July 1, 1988

Susan Alder   Gerhard Zbinden

A Look Behind Drug Regulatory Guidelines

G. Zbinden

1. Shortcomings of Guidelines for Drug Safety Testing

In the very beginning when formalized drug registration was in its infancy, some well-meaning scientists in regulatory agencies issued tentative instructions on how to go about toxicity testing of new drugs. I remember a set of slides shown by Arnold J. Lehman of the FDA at a Joint Symposium on Safety Evaluation of new Drugs, sponsored by the A.M.A. Section of Experimental Medicine and Therapeutics and the Society of Toxicology in Atlantic City N.J. on June 17, 1963. They were photographed by somebody and found their way through clandestine channels into every toxicology laboratory of the Unites States and beyond. These slides are reproduced on pages 15 to 19. A comparison with the modern guidelines described in this book demonstrates how much the concepts developed at the FDA some 30 years ago have influenced drug toxicology ever since.

Later, much more elaborate directions were issued, modestly called guidelines or notes for guidance. Those stemming from powerful national regulatory agencies or well-organized international bodies such as the EEC, WHO and the OECD, achieved a notoriety and prominence which put them well above the helpful hints and instructions that toxicologists needed to design meaningful experiments. As a matter of fact, some modern guidelines have become so detailed that they serve as testing protocols from which one does not lightly deviate.

Drug regulatory guidelines are very strange pieces of writing indeed. None has, to my knowledge, ever been published in a refereed scientific journal. At first sight, most of their content appears quite reasonable and straightforward. However, a closer look reveals stipulations that certainly have never been subjected to scientific scrutiny. Here are a few examples:

– «Experiments have to be done on two species one of which a non-rodent». One may ask why two species must be used, and not three or only one? Why not two rodents or two non-rodents?

– «Animals must be treated once daily and 7 days a week». This preposterous rule which is contrary to the elementary concepts of pharmacokinetics is found, with a few notable exceptions, in most regulatory guidelines.

– «The treatment should include: (a) a high dose selected for the purpose of causing target organ toxicity whenever possible or, failing this, other non-specific toxicity, or until limited by volume of dose; ...» (EEC, 1983). This idea that toxicity must be induced at all cost, even if one has to choke the animals with gram quantities of certain compounds, was probably also hatched at the offices of the FDA. The chief toxicologist, Arnold J. Lehman, wrote already in 1959: «Since it is generally accepted procedure to employ three dosage levels in such studies, one dosage level should be the toxic dose regardless of what multiple of the therapeutic dose may be required to obtain toxicity». No critical scientific examination of

General Comments

this practice has ever been conducted.

Reading drug regulatory guidelines, I am reminded of the instructions for the assembly of an outdoor barbecue rotisserie which the author of the incomparable book «Zen and the Art of Motorcycle Maintenance», Robert M. Pirsig, tried to explain to a couple of friends. I felt I have to include this part of the book here, and if you just substitute «toxicology» for «rotisserie», and «testing procedure» for «machine» you will understand why.

> «The rotisserie instructions begin and end exclusively with the machine. But the kind of approach I'am thinking about doesn't cut it off so narrowly. What's really angering about instructions of this sort is that they imply there's only one way to put this rotisserie together – *their* way. And that presumption wipes out all the creativity. Actually there are hundreds of ways to put the rotisserie together and when they make you follow just one way without showing you the overall problem the instructions become hard to follow in such a way as not to make mistakes. You loose feeling for the work. And not only that, it's very unlikely that they have told you the best way.»
>
> «But they're from the *factory*,» John says.
>
> «I'm from the factory too,» I say, «and I *know* how instructions like this are put together. You go out on the assembly line with a tape recorder and the foreman sends you to talk to the guy he needs least, the biggest goof-off he's got, and whatever he tells you – that's the instructions. The next guy might have told you something completely different and probably better, but he's too busy.»
>
> They all look surprised.
>
> «I might have known» DeWeese says.
>
> «It's the format,» I say. «No writer can buck it. Technology presumes there's just one right way to do things and there never is. And when you presume there's just one right way to do things, of *course* the instructions begin and end exclusively with the rotisserie. But if you have to choose among an infinite number of ways to put it together then the relation of the machine to you, and the relation of the machine and you to the rest of the world, has to be considered, because the selection from many choices, the *art* of the work is just as dependent upon your own mind and spirit as it is upon the material of the machine. That's why you need the peace of mind.»
>
> «Actually this idea isn't so strange,» I continue. «Sometime look at a novice workman or a bad workman and compare his expression with that of a craftsman whose work you know is excellent and you'll see the difference. The craftsman isn't ever following a single line of instruction. He's making decisions as he goes along. For that reason he'll be absorbed and attentive to what he's doing even though he doesn't deliberately contrive this. His motions and the machine are in a kind of harmony. He isn't following any set of written instructions because the nature of the material at hand determines his thoughts and motions, which simultaneously change the nature of the material at hand. The material and his thoughts are changing together in a progression of changes until his mind's at rest at the same time the material's right.»

«Sounds like art,» the instructor says.

«Well it *is* art,» I say. «This divorce of art from technology is completely unnatural. It's just that it's gone on so long you have to be an archeologist to find out where the two separated. Rotisserie assembly is actually a long-lost branch of sculpture, so divorced from its roots by centuries of intellectual wrong turns that just to associate the two sounds ludicrous.»

They're not sure whether I'm kidding or not.

«You mean,» DeWeese asks, «that when I was putting this rotisserie together I was actually sculpting it?»

«Sure».

He goes over this in his mind, smiling more and more. «I wish I'd known that,» he says. Laughter follows.

I was tempted to underline sentences that appeared to be particularly appropriate to my discussion of the shortcomings of toxicological guidelines, but when I started I found that most of them fell under this heading. However, if I had to select just one sentence that sums up my thoughts, it would be: «Technology presumes there's just one right way to do things and there never is.» Remember that toxicology deals with chemicals as diverse as drugs, pesticides, cosmetics, food additives, industrial chemicals and environmental pollutants. They not only differ widely with regard to chemical structure and physical properties, but span the whole spectrum of imaginable biological activities. How is it possible then that an identical approach and essentially the same testing protocols should be used to determine their toxicological characteristics? Are we really permitted to assume that there is only one right way to test for chemical toxicity?

2. When Guidelines Fail

It is undeniable that the very existence of detailed safety testing guidelines greatly facilitates the development process of new drugs. Since it takes years from the successful synthesis of a new chemical to its ultimate introduction as a new drug on the market, and since these years are filled with a vast and ever-increasing array of safety tests, it is convenient indeed to have binding instructions on how to perform toxicological studies in such a way that they will be acceptable to regulatory agencies many years hence. The more authoritative the guidelines, the better for the industrial toxicologist. The hundreds of other ways that could be devised to study the safety of new compounds may provide a stimulating intellectual exercise and lead to illuminating scientific discoveries, but if my snooping around the boundaries of standard toxicological practice provides findings that are unexplained or not acceptable to regulatory agencies, the development of a new drug may be greatly retarded and occasionally even aborted. So if I want to keep my job, I am better off doing toxicology *their* way and forgetting about creativity. And if I hope to market my drug on a worldwide basis, I am going to use the guidelines that are the most demanding with regard to numbers of species, subjects and dose levels, and duration of treatment. I can be sure that no regulatory agency will object to a toxicological dossier that is more voluminous than the one it might consider desirable or necessary.

General Comments

Fortunately, there are situations where regulatory requirements simply cannot be met. And suddenly, we realize what these guidelines really are: convenient instructions for the typical case, an easily enforceable manual that relieves me of the burden of creating a new set of testing rules for each compound, the antithesis of the famous «case by case approach» toxicologists sometimes dream about.

Let me mention a few instances where official drug testing requirements cannot be fulfilled: conventional fertility studies cannot be performed with contraceptive agents, and standard rules for teratogenicity tests are not applicable for abortifacients. In vitro mutagenicity experiments with antibiotics using bacteria are often not possible, and equally erratic results are obtained in mutagenicity tests with mammalian cells, if the test compounds are highly cytotoxic. For all in vitro experiments, poor solubility of the test substance in water is an obstacle that is often unsurmountable (although some people do not seem to mind if their cells and bacteria must swim between the prickly crystals of undissolved test chemicals).

Meaningful repeated-dose toxicity studies are hardly possible with drugs having potent and life-threatening pharmacodynamic actions, as we have once demonstrated with strychnine (Seidl and Zbinden, 1982) and as it becomes evident in toxicity studies with drugs causing intestinal paralysis. Another example is provided by postnatal toxicity tests with substances that inhibit the flow of milk. Sometimes, toxic responses preclude performance of valid safety tests, a typical case being the marked ulcerogenic effects of nonsteroidal antiinflammatory and antineoplastic drugs. Some compounds cause vomiting in dogs, and any attempt to administer such drugs by the oral route is thwarted by the animal's violent reflexes.

Quite often, test chemicals, even drugs, prove to be so innocuous that a dose causing overt signs of toxicity simply cannot be reached. There are many reasons for this, e.g. poor bioavailability, extensive first-pass metabolism, rapid renal clearance or lack of intrinsic toxicity. The concern that regulatory agencies might not accept a toxicity test in which no toxic dose was reached, sometimes incites the toxicologists to resort to grotesque overdosing, a practice that is not only cruel to the animals but bound to produce meaningless results.

Quite often, drugs are not stable at acidic pH and must, therefore, be administered as an enteric coated formulation. A similar galenic dosage form can often be made for toxicity studies in dogs and other large animals, but is usually not practical for experiments in small rodents. There are many other galenic formulations specially prepared for use in humans, e.g. drug-loaded devices such as intrauterine loops and vaginal rings, transdermal applicators, suppositories and slow-release capsules. In many instances, the geometry and size of these objects make it impossible to design toxicity studies in which the mode of application corresponds to that envisaged for clinical use. Another major problem is posed by the testing of drugs administered by inhalation, since it is impossible to incite an animal to inhale so deeply that the drug will reach the alveoles.

In recent years, two new developments in therapy and diagnostics have pitilessly revealed the shortcomings of classical drug regulatory guidelines: namely, biomaterials, i.e. the many polymers that are used as implants and prosthetic devices, and the products of biotechnology such as human proteins and peptides obtained by recombinant DNA procedures and their semisynthetic derivatives, synthetic peptides and monoclonal antibodies. The biomaterials open up whole new areas of toxicological concern (Zbinden, 1986), and the products of biotechnology defy our best efforts to investigate their safety by inducing laboratory animals to make antibodies directed against the test compounds. Moreover, toxic responses to these agents seen in humans are often not present in animals since their organs lack the necessary receptors (Zbinden, 1987).

One can, of course, try to apply the standard guidelines even in those cases in which the futility of the approach is blatantly evident. I have mentioned a typical case before, the drugs that fail to induce toxicity even at high doses. As I also mentioned, some drug regulatory agencies still insist that such compounds be given in amounts that induce non-specific toxicity or, failing even this, that the doses be increased until limited by the sheer volume that can be forced down the throat of the helpless laboratory animal (EEC, 1983). I hope that stipulations of this kind will soon be eliminated from all drug regulatory guidelines, and that current standards of pharmacokinetics will finally also be applied to drug safety testing (Zbinden, 1988).

How should we proceed if standard regulatory guidelines simply cannot be followed, what alternatives are left? I have tried to give a simple anwer to this difficult question in what I once called the «second law of toxicology» which runs thus: «When standard toxicological procedures and regulatory guidelines cannot be applied, do the best you can». Instead of working by the book, we must proceed in the same way as the craftsman-artist, decribed by Pirsig:

«The craftsman isn't ever following a single line of instruction. He's making decisions as he goes along. For that reason he'll be absorbed and attentive to what he's doing even though he doesn't deliberately contrive this. His motions and the machine are in a kind of harmony. He isn't following any set of written instructions because the nature of the material at hand determines his thoughts and motions, which simultaneously change the nature of the material at hand».

In experimental toxicology, this mode of operation goes by the name of «case by case approach». It always starts with an analysis of the problem and attempts to predict, on a theoretical basis, the potential human hazards that could be associated with the use of the compound or material at hand. It then describes the shortcomings of the available standard testing models for the particular problem, and proposes feasible alternative procedures that can contribute to the assessment of the potential human hazards identified initially. Thus, one attempts to come up with a set of partial answers, that, when taken together, are more valuable than a technically deficient standard test.

3. Animal Welfare

Many of the toxicological test procedures inflict substantial pain and anxiety on the laboratory animals. This is particularly true for animals used in acute toxicity studies, and those included in the high dose groups of repeated-dose experi-

General Comments

ments. Considerable suffering must be assumed in animals bearing large tumors or afflicted with organ damage, e.g. perforated gastrointestinal ulcers, myocardial infarctions, liver necrosis and muscle wasting. Functional disturbances such as paralysis, excessive central nervous system stimulation, diarrhea, polyuria, hypotension and sensory organ dysfunction cause stress and anxiety. Repeated injections often induce considerable local pain, and animals sometimes struggle desperately to avoid another injection. Topical administration of irritant and corrosive substances to the skin and mucous membranes is a painful procedure that has come under particularly heavy criticism by animal welfare advocates.

A look at regulatory guidelines for safety studies shows that they are essentially silent on the animal welfare issues. A notable exception is the proposed revision of the OECD[1] Guideline for Testing of Chemicals 401, Acute Oral Toxicity of April 11, 1986. It includes the following statement: «Animals showing severe and enduring signs of distress and pain may need to be humanely killed. Doses known to cause marked pain and distress, due to corrosive or severely irritant actions, need not be administered, even when no mortality has been observed at tolerated doses.» Although I would have preferred to see the «may need» and «need» replaced by «must», I am pleased that a modest first step in favor of animal welfare has been made in a guideline of a highly reputable international organization.

The pain and anxiety of laboratory animals is first and foremost an ethical issue that deserves to be acknowledged in official regulations that deal with the performance of safety tests on live animals. Binding instructions on when to discontinue treatment and when to kill animals that suffer or are irreparably damaged should be part of every drug safety guideline. It must also be acknowledged that the experimental results may be compromised or invalidated if the treatment puts the animals under heavy stress. It certainly cannot be the purpose of toxicological investigations to produce data that cannot be interpreted owing to the poor general conditions and the severe disarray of all vital functions of the subjects.

In many countries new animal welfare legislation has been enacted or is under discussion, and clearly these laws could potentially influence our way of conducting drug safety studies. It is equally evident that animal protection laws will occasionally come into direct conflict with official rules of drug safety testing.

A common feature of many new animal protection laws is the requirement to demonstrate the advisability, in some countries even the unconditional necessity, of all proposed animal experiments. It is probable that those reviewing applications for toxicological studies will expect more justification for an animal experiment than the simple statement that the proposed test is necessary because it is required by a regulatory guideline. In particular, permission to conduct a toxicological experiment will not easily be obtained if the country in which the study will be conducted does not require the proposed test, or is satisfied with an experiment involving fewer animals or a shorter duration of treatment. Thus, the easy way out described above, i.e. to conduct toxicity studies always according to the most demanding national guideline, will, in the future, often not be possible. As a consequence, the national drug safety testing guidelines described in this book, will become of much greater importance than they were only a few years ago. On the other hand, stricter control of toxicity studies on the national level carries the

General Comments

risk that some of the data obtained in one country may not be acceptable in others. In the light of these developments, a critical review of the aims, approaches and protocols of drug toxicity testing will have to be undertaken, and a renewed effort must be made to harmonize the national guidelines so that the smallest number of animals possible is used to obtain generally acceptable toxicological information. The international effort to reassess and redesign the procedures for acute toxicity testing which has led to a dramatic reduction of animal use, should provide sound directions for this important task.

---

1) the OECD guidelines are not primarily intended for drugs and are not part of this collection.

References

EEC (1983) Notes for guidance concerning the application of chapter I(B)(2) of part 2 of the Annex to Directive 75/318/EEC, with the view of the granting of a marketing authorization for a new drug. Official Journal of the European Communities, 28.11.83.

Lehman, A.J. (1959) Newer trends in laboratory evaluation of the safety of drugs. Bull. of the Parent. Drug Assoc. 13: 2-6.

Seidl, I., and Zbinden, G. (1982) Subchronic oral toxicity of strychnine in rats. Arch. Toxicol. 51: 267-272.

Zbinden, G. (1988) Biopharmaceutical studies, a key to better toxicology. Xenobiotica 18, Suppl. 1: 3-7.

Zbinden, G. (1987) Biotechnology products for human use, toxicological targets and strategies. In: Preclinical Safety of Biotechnology Products for Human Use. Charles E. Graham, ed. Alan R. Liss Inc. New York, pp 143-159.

Zbinden, G. (1986) Zur toxikologischen Prüfung von Biomaterialien. In: Aktuelle Probleme der Biomedizin, O.K. Burger, P. Grosdanoff, D. Henschler, O. Kraupp. B. Schniders, eds. Walter de Gruyter & Co, Berlin, pp 305-313.

Slides shown with talk by A.J. Lehman, M.D. «The Intent of the Preclinical Assessment of New Drugs» at Joint Symposium on Safety Evaluation of New Drugs. Sponsored by A.M.A. Sect. of Exper. Med. & Therap. and the Society of Toxicology, Atlantic City, N.J. June 17, 1963.

SLIDE 1

Route: oral or parenteral

Phase I.

(A) As a single dose of not more than for a few days in any one individual.
Acute toxicity: 4 species, one a non-rodent.
Subacute toxicity: 2 species, one a non-rodent, at 3 dosage levels for 2 weeks.
Clinical laboratory tests:
  Hemograms in both species, including coagulation tests.
  Liver function in both species (SGPT).
  Alkaline phosphatase in non-rodent only.
  Kidney function in non-rodent only.
  Fasting blood sugar in both species.
Histopathology: Gross and microscopic studies of major organs and others if indicated.
Special study: Irritation studies if parenteral.

SLIDE 2

Phase II.

(A) Single administration clinically (diagnostic drugs, local anesthetics). No further studies beyond Phase I.

(B) Initial clinical trial of 1 to 2 weeks.
Subacute toxicity: 2 species, one a non-rodent, at 3 dosage levels for 4 weeks.
Histopathology: Gross and microscopic examination in considerable detail.

(C) One to 3 months clinical trial.
No further observations beyond (B) above.

(D) 6 months to unlimited trial.
Subacute toxicity: 2 species, one a non-rodent, at 3 dosage levels for 3 months.

SLIDE 3

Phase III:

(A) Large-scale clinical trial of a single dose.
No further studies beyond Phase I.

(B) 2 weeks clinical trial.
Subacute toxicity: 2 species, one a non-rodent, at 3 dosage levels for up to 90 days depending upon the particular situation.

(C) One to 3 months clinical trial.
Subacute toxicity: As above but extended to 90 days.

(D) 6 months to unlimited clinical trial.
Subacute toxicity: 2 species, one a non-rodent, at 3 dosage levels for at least 6 months, and extended to 1 to 1 1/2 years in rats and 2 to 3 years in dogs.

SLIDE 4

Route: general anesthetics by inhalation

Phase I.

Subacute toxicity:
4 species including those known to be sensitive to related drugs.
Administer anesthetic for 3 hours continuously on 5 consecutive days under conditions of clinical use.
Other observations as for oral and parenteral drugs.
Histopathology: Lungs, liver, adrenal, kidney, thyroid, and others if sugggested by abnormal response (e.g. CNS).

Phase II.
No further observations beyond Phase I.

Phase III.
No further observations beyond Phase I.

SLIDE 5

> Route: dermal
>
> Phase I.
>
> > Acute toxicity: 2 species, one a non-rodent, orally.
> > Special study: Acute dermal (single exposure) for 24 hours. Minimal observation period of 2 weeks. Blood and urine are examined, and body weight, food consumption, and behavior are recorded.
> > Histopathology: Gross inspection of viscers, and microscopic studies as indicated.
>
> Phase II.
>
> > Subacute toxicity: 20-day dermal toxicity on intact and abraded skin at 1, 3, and 10 times human dose on a body-weight basis.
> > Histopathology: Gross and microscopic study of skin and other organs as indicated.
>
> Phase III.
>
> (A) Short-term clinical trial.
> No further studies beyond Phase II.
>
> (B) Unlimited trial.
> Phase II is extended to include a 90-day study on intact skin.

SLIDE 6

> Route: ophthalmic
>
> Phase I.
>
> > Acute toxicity: 2 species, one a non-rodent, orally.
> > Special study: Irritation study on single exposure at several concentrations and dosage levels (constant volume) employing the rabbit eye.
> > No furhter studies required.
>
> Phase II.
>
> > Subacute toxicity: 3 weeks daily applications (must be repeated several times daily if so used in practice).
> > Histopathology: On eyes and adnexa that exhibit gross or slit lamp changes.
>
> Phase III.
>
> > No further studies needed beyond Phase II.

SLIDE 7

> Route: vaginal or rectal
>
> Phase I.
>
> > Acute toxicity: 2 species, one a non-rodent, orally.
> >
> > Special study: Local and systemic toxicity by single vaginal or rectal administration in the rat and non-rodent.
>
> Phase II.
>
> > Subacute toxicity: Daily administration by the appropriate route at several dosage levels in a single species. Duration and number of applications are determined by proposed clinical use.
> >
> > Clinical laboratory tests: Hematology and clinical chemistry as may be indicated.
> >
> > Histopathology: Gross and microscopic examination of mucous membrane involved, and other tissues and organs as may be indicated.
>
> Phase III.
>
> > No further studies beyond Phase II.

SLIDE 8

> Combination of 2 or more drugs where toxicity data are available on each drug individually
>
> Phase I.
>
> > Acute toxicity: LD50 determination (whenever possible by the recommended route clinically) of the combination in the rat compared to individual concurrent LD50's for indication of possible potentiation.
>
> Phase II.
>
> > Acute toxicity: LD50 of the combination as given above.
> >
> > Subacute toxicity: A 30 to 90-day study in rats and dogs on the combination by the route recommended clinically. Duration will depend upon the particular situation and will have to be individualized.
> >
> > Clinical laboratory studies: As given in Phase I for oral and parenteral drugs.
> >
> > Histopathology: Gross and microscopic studies in considerable detail.

SLIDE 9

Phase III.

    Nor further studies beyond Phase II.

    If the combination consists of 2 or more drugs without adequate toxicity data available, «sliding scale» procedure may be tried. The $LD50$'s of various combinations should be determined in the rat and compared to individual concurrent $LD50$'s of the drugs as determined individually.

European Economic Community (EEC)

Documents reviewed:

EEC I: Official Journal of the European Communities, No. L 147 (75/318/EEC), June 9, 1975. Council Directive of 20 May 1975 on the approximation of the laws of Member States relating to analytical, pharmacotoxicological and clinical standards and protocols in respect of the testing of proprietary medicinal products.
EEC II: Official Journal of the European Communities, No. L 332 (83/571/EEC), November 28, 1983. Council recommendation of 26 October 1983 concerning tests relating to the placing on the market of proprietary medicinal products.
EEC III: Official Journal of the European Communities, No. L 15 (87/19/EEC, amending directive 75/318/EEC), January 17, 1987. Council directive of 22 December 1986 amending Directive 75/318/EEC on the approximation of the laws of the Member States relating to analytical, pharmaco-toxicological and clinical standards and protocols in respect of the testing of proprietary medicinal products.
EEC IV: Official Journal of the European Communities, No. L 73 (87/176/EEC), March 16, 1987. Council recommendation of 9 February 1987 concerning tests relating to the placing on the market of proprietary medicinal products.
For details on presentation of application consult **EEC V**, not summarized below (no legal force):
EEC V: Notice to Applicants for Marketing Authorizations for Proprietary Medicinal Products in the Member States of the EC. Final Draft, June, 1987.

Address of Regulatory Agency:

Commission of the European Communities, Directorate-General for Internal Market and Industrial Affairs, Rue de la Loi 200, B-1049 Brussels, Belgium.

Summary of Toxicological Guidelines:

EEC I: Official Journal of the European Communities, No. L 147 (75/318(EEC), June 9, 1975. Council Directive of 20 May 1975 on the approximation of the laws of Member States relating to analytical, pharmacotoxicological and clinical standards and protocols in respect of the testing of proprietary medicinal products.

Single dose toxicity (acute toxicity)

Species:	At least 2 mammalian of known strain.
Sex:	Equal numbers of M and F.
Route:	At least 2, one of which identical with or similar to that proposed for use in man, one ensuring systemic absorption of substance.
Determination of LD50:	Where possible with its fiducial limits (95 %).

EEC

Observation period:	To be fixed by the investigator, not less than one week.
Variables:	Signs, including local reactions.
Combinations:	In the case of active substances in combination, study must be carried out in such a way as to check whether or not potentiation or novel toxic effects occur.
Note:	These guidelines are now replaced by revised guidelines described under EEC IV, page 30.

Repeated dose toxicity (sub-acute or chronic toxicity)

Species:	2 mammalian, one a non-rodent.
Duration:	Generally 2 tests: one short-term, lasting 2-4 weeks; one long-term, lasting 3-6 months, depending on conditions of clinical use. For drugs given to humans only once: 2-4 weeks.
Frequency of administration:	To be clearly stated.
Dose levels:	Reasons for dosages chosen to be given. Maximum dose to be chosen so as to bring harmful effects to light. Lower dose will then enable the animals' tolerance of the product to be determined.
Route:	Choice of routes shall depend on intended therapeutic use and possibilities of systemic absorption.
Experimental procedure:	Wherever possible, and always in experiments on small rodents, design of experiment and control procedures must be suited to the scale of the problem being tackled and enable fiducial limits to be determined.
Variables:	Behavior, growth, hematological and biochemical tests, especially those relating to the excretory mechanism, autopsy reports, histological data.
Method:	Choice and range of each group of tests will depend on species of animal used and the state of scientific knowledge at the time.
Combinations:	In the case of new combinations of known substances that have been investigated in accordance with the provisions of this Directive, long-term tests may, except where acute and subacute toxicity tests have demonstrated potentiation or novel toxic effects, be modified by investigator who shall submit his reasons for such modification. Substances that have been shown to be safe by wide usage over at least 3 years in clinical treatment of human beings, and by the results of controlled trials shall be treated in the same way as known substances which have already been investigated in accordance with these standards and protocols.
Excipient:	An excipient used for the first time shall be treated like an active ingredient.
Note:	These guidelines are extended: See EEC II, page 24.

EEC

Fetal toxicity

Omission of these tests must be adequately justified.

Species: At least 2: a breed of rabbits sensitive to known teratogenic substances and rats or mice (specifying the strain) or, if appropriate, some other animal species.
Number
of animals:
Dose levels: shall depend on state of scientific knowledge at the time
Timing when the application is lodged, and level of statistical sig-
of administration: nificance that results must attain.
Variables:
Note: These guidelines are amplified in EEC II, p 24.

Reproduction study

If results of other tests reveal anything suggesting harmful effects on progeny or impairment of M or F reproductive function, this shall be investigated by appropriate tests.

Note: These guidelines are now extended. See EEC II, p 24.

Carcinogenicity:

Requirements: – Substances having a close chemical analogy with known carcinogenic or co-carcinogenic compounds.
– Substances which have given rise to suspicious changes during long-term toxicological tests.
– Substances which have given rise to suspicious results in mutagenic-potential tests or in other short-term carcinogenicity tests.
– Substances to be included in proprietary medicinal products likely to be administered regularly over a prolonged period of a patients's life.
Method: According to the state of scientific knowledge at the time when the application is lodged.
Note: These guidelines are amplified in EEC II, p 24.

Mutagenicity

Requirements: Obligatory for any new substance.
Method: Number and types of tests and criteria for their evaluation shall depend on the state of scientific knowledge at the time when the application is lodged.

Local toxicity

Requirement: Where a proprietary medicinal product is intended for topical use.
Scope of study: Investigation of systemic absorption of product, also for possible use on broken skin.
Method: If systemic absorption under these conditions is negligible,

repeated dose systemic toxicity tests, fetal toxicity tests and studies of reproductive function may be omitted.

If systemic absorption is demonstrated during therapeutic experimentation, toxicity tests shall be carried out on animals, and where necessary, fetal toxicity tests.

In all cases tests of local tolerance after repeated application shall be carried out and include histological examinations. Possibility of sensitization shall be investigated and any carcinogenic potential.

EEC II: Official Journal of the European Communities, No. L 332 (83/571/EEC), November 28, 1983. Council recommendation of 26 October 1983 concerning tests relating to the placing on the market of proprietary medicinal products.

Repeated dose toxicity

Species:	At least 2, one a non-rodent, to be chosen on the basis of their similarity to man.
Sex:	Equal numbers of M and F.
Duration:	According to proposed duration of human treatment.

in man:	in animal:
– 1 or repeated doses in 1 day	2 weeks
– up to 7 days	4 weeks
– up to 30 days	3 months
– beyond 30 days or intermittently with total of 1 month or more in a year, or when retention is prolonged	6 months

Note: The use of a 4 week test as a range finding study is recommended.

Frequency of administration:	7 days per week. Less frequently when rate of elimination slow. More than once per day if rate of elimination fast or gastric intolerance present.
Route:	That intended for use in man (if technically possible). Pharmacological effects should be demonstrable. If not, other routes should be considered.
Dose levels:	3. – High dose causing target organ toxicity or non-specific toxicity or until limited by volume. – Low dose: sufficient to produce pharmacodynamic effect or therapeutic effect or blood levels comparable to those expected to produce these effects in man. – Intermediate dose, such as geometric mean between high and low dose.
Control groups:	Appropriate control groups, positive controls if necessary.
Size of groups:	No exact numbers are given. Consideration to be given: to obtain all toxicologically relevant effects, to permit interim sacrifices and reversibility studies. – Size limited for practical and financial reasons and for humane considerations.
Variables:	Food intake, body weight, hematology, clinical chemistry, urinalysis, ophthalmology, ECG, general behavior.
Autopsy:	All animals.
Histopathology:	– Rodents: all organs and tissues of high dose and control groups. Lower dose groups only for organs and tissues showing pathological changes at autopsy. – Non-rodents: all animals of all doses. Tissues to be studied histologically: Gross lesions, tissue masses or tumors (including regional

	lymph nodes), blood smears (in case of anemia, enlarged thymus, lymphadenopathy), lymph nodes, mammary glands, salivary glands, sternebrae, femur or vertebrae (including bone marrow), pituitary, thymus, trachea, lungs, heart, thyroid, esophagus, stomach, small intestine (Swiss roll method), colon, liver, gall-bladder, pancreas, spleen, kidneys, adrenals, bladder, prostate, testes, ovaries, uterus, brain (coronal sections at three levels), eyes, spinal cord.
Immuno-interference:	According to the actual state of knowledge.

Inhalation studies

Requirements:	Where: a) pharmacokinetics after administration by inhalation may differ qualitatively or quantitatively from the pattern after other routes of administration b) drug and propellant may interact in the body c) the inhaled product may have a local effect in the airways, either a short-term or a long term effect.
Species:	At least one rodent and one non-rodent for repeated exposure studies. Animals should be free of pulmonary infection and have low incidence of other pulmonary pathology.
Number of animals:	Number in each group should be adequate for statistical analysis and will be determined by duration of experiment and by number of observations, measurements and interim sacrifices.
Duration:	Should be related to some extent to proposed human exposure.
Administration:	Depends on nature of substance and intended use in man. In acute studies reasonable to administer substance directly into airways via nasotracheal tube or through tracheotomy. In long-term studies «head only» or «nose only» exposure chambers or masks for inhalation necessary. If whole body exposure is used, deposition of drug on skin, in pelt, in upper airways and amount swallowed should be taken into account in determining dose of substance administered. It should be demonstrated that method of administration ensures that substance reaches the desired site.
Dose levels:	Normally 3. In selection of dose levels same principles should apply as for toxicity studies by other routes. Different levels of drug exposure achieved by alteration of concentration of substance or by alteration of duration of exposure.
Controls:	One or more, as appropriate.

EEC

Reproduction study

Requirement:	All new drugs.
Scope of study:	– Changes in fertility or in the production of abnormal young due to damage to the M and/or F gametes – interference with pre-implantation and implantation stages in the development of the conceptus – toxic effects on the embryo – toxic effects on the fetus – changes in maternal physiology producing secondary effects on embryo or fetus – effects on uterine or placental growth or development – interference with parturition – effects on postnatal development and suckling of the progeny and on maternal lactation – late effects on the progeny.
Type of study:	No rigid requirements. Choice of studies to be justified by investigator.
Species:	2 mammalian, one a non-rodent for embryotoxicity studies. For fertility and perinatal studies at least one. Desirabale, that one of the species is same as in long-term toxicity studies.
Administration:	– Embryotoxicity: throughout period of embryogenesis. – Fertility study: sufficient time before mating to reveal drug effect on gametogenesis. In rodents: M at least 60 days F at least 14 days prior to mating, throughout pregnancy. Dosed animals may be mated with dosed partners. If positive effects obtained experiment must be repeated with undosed partners. – Perinatal studies: from end of organogenesis up to weaning.
Route:	That proposed in man.
Dose levels:	3. – Highest dose to cause some maternal toxicity, e.g. decrease in body weight gain. – Low dose to produce pharmacodynamic effect similar to desired therapeutic effect or to produce blood levels comparable to those required to produce the effect. (Exception: this does not apply if pharmacodynamic effect by itself causes toxicity.) – Intermediate dose: geometric mean of high and low dose.
Number of animals:	With exception of primates, the following minimum number of animals suggested:

EEC

	– Embryotoxicity studies: 20 pregnant F in rodents, 12 pregnant F in non-rodents per dose level. – Fertility studies: 24 F and 24 M per dose level. – Perinatal studies: 12 pregnant F per dose level.
Housing and diet:	Details to be given.
Pharmacokinetics:	Level of exposure of fetus to be determined.
Variables:	– Embryotoxicity studies: number of corpora lutea, implantation sites, resorptions, weight and sex of fetuses, external abnormalities, skeleton or viscera. – Fertility studies: F killed during gestation: as above. F allowed to litter: number of pups should be allowed to reach maturity. In these auditory, visual and behavioral impairment should be assessed. Reproductive function in at least 1 M and 1 F from each litter (no brother/sister mating). – Pre- and postnatal dosing: autopsy at weaning. Unter certain circumstances progeny may be allowed to live to maturity so that reproductive capacity can be assessed. In these determination of behavioral, visual and auditory impairment.

Carcinogenicity

Requirements:	– Drug administered over a substantial period of life, e.g. continuously during a minimum period of 6 months, or frequently in intermittent manner so that total exposure is similar. – Chemical structure suggesting carcinogenic potential. – Belonging to therapeutic class with members having given carcinogenic results. – Its pattern of toxicity or long-term retention detected in previous studies. – Positive findings in mutagenicity and short-term carcinogenicity studies. – Not required for drug used exclusively in patients with short life expectancy. – Insoluble substances which are not absorbed may not require carcinogenicity tests.
Species:	2, preferably those with metabolism of drug similar to man. Species and strains with high incidence of spontaneous tumors should be avoided. Species and strains should be known to be sensitive to one or more carcinogens.
Sex:	M and F.
Age:	As soon as possible after weaning.
Duration:	Rats: 24 months, mice and hamsters: 18 months. Where survival rate is high, rats: 30 months, mice: 24 months, or lifespan of animal, i.e. to 20 % survival in controls.

EEC

Administration:	Daily.
Route:	That proposed in man.
Dose levels:	3.

– High dose: to produce minimum toxic effects, e.g. a 10 % weight loss, or failure to grow, or minimal target organ toxicity.
– Low dose: 2 to 3 times the maximum human therapeutic dose or that which produces a pharmacological effect.
– Intermediate dose: geometric mean of high and low dose. Exception: toxic dose is a high multiple of therapeutic dose. In this case high dose = 100 times human therapeutic dose.

Number of animals:	For routine tests with mice, rats, hamsters, 50 of each sex per treated group.
Controls:	2 control groups of 50 per dose and sex. Positive control groups not required.
Diet:	Specifications to be provided.
Autopsy:	All animals.
Histopathology:	All tissues listed of all high dose animals and all controls. Tissues with macroscopic lesions, tissues and organs found to have tumors with high dose: middle and low dose groups should also be examined.
Tissues:	Same as in repeated-dose toxicity studies, see p 25.
Analysis of data:	Statistical procedures used should be clearly stated. The responses should be assessed in following ways:

Total incidence of tumor bearing animals and of tumors. Incidence of tumors involving a specific tissue, and those judged to be malignant. Latent period to tumor appearance.
Analysis should be directed towards assessment of:
– presence of any effect of substance, as shown by contrast between response in the 3 treatment groups, as a set, and in the 2 control groups, as a set
– whether any effect is dose-related, as shown by a trend in the responses in low-, mid- and high-dose groups.
Professional statistical advice should be available in order to assess influence of other factors (death of test animals because of other diseases, premature killing of animals because of clinical detection of tumors).
Different circumstances may result in:
– an increased incidence or reduced latency of malignant tumors
– an increased incidence of benign tumors
– local induction of tumors at the site of injection.

EEC III: Official Journal of the European Communities, No. L 15 (87/19/EEC, amending Directive 75/318/EEC), January 17, 1987. Council Directive of 22 December 1986 amending Directive 75/318/EEC on the approximation of the laws of the Member States relating to analytical, pharmaco-toxicological and clinical standards and protocols in respect of the testing of proprietary medicinal products.

Acute toxicity, amendments

Species:	At least 2 mammalian of known strain **unless a single species can be justified**.
Sex:	**(not mentioned)**
Observation period:	To be fixed by the investigator, **usually 14 days**, but not less than one week, **but without exposing animals to prolonged suffering.**
Determination of LD50:	**Quantitative evaluation of approximate LD and information on dose-effect relationship should be obtained, but high level of precision is not required.**
Method:	**The maximum amount of information should be obtained from the animals used in study**

EEC IV: Official Journal of the European Communities, No. L 73 (87/176/EEC), March 16, 1987. Council recommendation of 9 February 1987 concerning tests relating to the placing on the market of proprietary medicinal products.

Single dose toxicity (acute toxicity studies)

Drug substances:	If possible same composition (e.g. pattern of impurities) as that proposed for marketing. In large animals testing of pharmaceutical formulation desirable. New excipients to be treated like new drug. In case of combination of active substances study of each active substance separately necessary, as well as testing of combination in same proportion as proposed in final product. In special cases consideration should be given to possible toxicity of degradation products.
Species:	At least 2 of known strain.
Sex:	Equal numbers of M and F. If no difference in response between M and F of first rodent species, only one sex to be used in other acute toxicity studies.
Administration:	Details, e.g. vehicle, adjuvants, concentrations, volume, pH etc. to be provided.
Route:	Rodents at least 2, one of which same as that proposed in man, one that ensures full access of unchanged drug into circulation. If use in man i.v. no other route necessary.
Dose levels:	Such that spectrum of toxicity is revealed.
Determination of LD:	Rodents for quantitative estimate of approximate LD and dose-effect relationship. High level of precision not required.
Observation period:	14 days or as long as signs of toxicity persist.
Experimental details:	E.g. age, sex, weight, origin, time of adaptation, SPF, vaccinations, homing, environmental conditions, diet etc. to be provided.
Autopsy:	All surviving animals and all animals dying during experiment.
Variables:	Signs of toxicity, time of occurrence, time and mode of death. Histopathology of any organ showing macroscopic changes.

Mutagenicity

Requirements:	Procedure should – be able to identify chemicals with mutagenic properties with maximum accuracy at reasonable cost – be capable of detecting main classes of genetic damage (gene, chromosome, genome mutations) – take into account that, although DNA is universal to prokaryotes and eukaryotes, the organization of genetic material is different.
Methods:	In vitro procedures and one in vivo test. According to specific characteristics of substance one of the

following 4 categories of tests should be selected (reason for selection to be justified by investigator):

a) Test for gene mutations in bacteria

Strains: Several well established strains.
Test methods: Tests to be carried out with and without extrinsic metabolic activation.

b) Test for chromosomal aberrations in mammalian cells in vitro

Cells: Human lymphocytes and several mammalian cell lines.
Test method: Tests to be carried out with and without extrinsic metabolic activation.
Variables: Damage scored by microscopic examination of chromosomes at mitotic metaphase.

c) Test for gene mutations in eukaryotic systems

Species / cells: Mammalian cells designed to detect induction of mutations at specific loci such as the ones coding for the enzymes hypoxanthine-guanine-phosphoribosyl-transferase or thymidine kinase. Other eukaryotes, such as fungi, insects may be considered.

d) In vivo test for genetic damage

Scope of study: To ascertain if a mutagenic compound has been missed by the in vitro tests because of inappropriate metabolic activation systems having been used. Best validated tests: those which have end points of chromosomal damage e.g. bone marrow metaphase and micronucleus tests and dominant lethal test. For somatic gene mutations: mouse spot test recommended.

Note: No test recommended for the detection of genome mutation, because specific methods presently under development are not sufficiently validated to incorporate them.
Above guidelines a)-d) under development, need to be periodically updated.

Interpretation of results: If all results indicate that substance has no effect in any of the tests then possibility of mutagenic hazard low. If all results both in vitro and in vivo indicate that compound has mutagenic properties then existence of a risk for humans high. If results are non-uniform significance of results to be judged not by their number but by their nature. Manufacturer should decide whether supplementary tests should be carried out and which ones. Selection of tests to be based on results already obtained as well as on other properties of compound and its intended use.

Risk consideration: Overall risk/benefit assessment should take into consideration: results of mutagenicity testing, pharmacokinetics, metabolism, and the whole toxicity profile. In addition, the intended use of the medicinal product, its degree of exposure, age and reproductive status of patient. Aspect of potential risk of alternatively available substances has to be taken into consideration.

NORDIC GUIDELINES
Denmark, Finland, Iceland, Norway and Sweden

Document reviewed:

NORTHERN COUNTRIES: Drug applications. Nordic guidelines. Prepared by Nordic Council on Medicines in cooperation with the Drug Regulatory Authorities in Denmark, Finland, Iceland, Norway, Sweden. NLN Publication No 12, Nordiska Läkemedelsnämnden. 1st edition, Uppsala November 1983.

Addresses of Regulatory Agencies:

DENMARK: Sundhedsstyrelsens farmaceutiske laboratorium, Frederikssundsvey 378, DK-2700 Bronshoj, Denmark.
FINLAND: Lääkintöhallitus/Medicinalstyrelsen, Apteekkitoimisto/Apoteksbyran, Siltasaarenkatu 18 A, PL 224, SF-00531 Helsinki 53, Finland.
ICELAND: Heilbrigdis- og Tryggingamalaraduneytid, Lyfjanefnd, Laugavegur 116, IS-105 Reykjavik, Iceland.
NORWAY: Statens legemiddelkontroll, Sven Oftedals vei 6, N-0950 Oslo, Norway.
SWEDEN: Socialstyrelsen läkemedelsavdelning, Box 607, S-751 25 Uppsala, Sweden.

Summary of Toxicological Guidelines:

Single dose toxicity

Species:	At least 2 suitable species.
Sex:	In certain cases M and F.
Route:	Various modes of administration.
Dose levels:	Concentration of the active substance in the preparation should be stated, as well as injection rate of i.v. formulations.
Determination of LD50:	Quantitative evaluation, though high level of precision not required. In addition to LD50 in rodents, highest tolerated dose and/or lowest lethal dose for other species, e.g. dog and rabbit, desirable.
Observation period:	7 days or longer, should be stated.
Variables:	Survival time of animals, toxic effects and time of their appearance, changes in animal's behavior and appearance, mode of death.
	Specification of species, strain, sex, age, weight, diet and any other conditions which may influence the result.
Experimental detail:	For drugs which may be used during the perinatal period,

33

data on acute toxicity in newborn animals should also be provided.

Repeated dose toxicity

Species:	At least 2, one non-rodent.
Dose levels:	At least 3.
Control groups:	Concurrent control groups and value of reference groups must be considered.
Reversibility:	Study of reversibility of observed toxic effects may be useful.
Variables:	Scope and frequency to be judged from case to case: Weight control, food and fluid intake, behavior and appearance, mortality (cause of death), hematology, blood chemistry, serum concentrations of the drug, functional investigations, e.g. ECG, neurological tests, ophthalmological examination, blood coagulation, urinalyses, macroscopic examinations, weights of organs, histopathology of organs and tissues with special emphasis on suspected target organs and organs of abnormal weight and appearance.
Special remarks:	For special dosage forms certain deviations from these recommendations may be appropriate.
Local effects:	Tests for drugs mainly intended to produce local effects (preparations for dermal, conjunctival, nasal, vaginal, rectal, and intra-articular application) should yield information about the drug's direct action on the relevant tissues. Special attention should be paid to data on absorption to determine whether or not the drug may have systemic effects. If systemic effects are likely to arise, performance of chronic toxicity test with oral or parenteral administration advisable. Duration of local toxicity test should be in reasonable proportion to that in clinical use.
Duration:	Depending on proposed use in man and intended duration of human exposure. Proposed repeated dose toxicity studies are listed below. In the case of discontinuous administration to humans of one month or more in one year, or when retention in the body of a single dose is prolonged, toxicity studies should last for at least 6 months.

1. Short term toxicity testing (subacute toxicity)

Species:	2 or more.
Exposure time:	For exposure to man of 1 to 7 days, minimum of 2 to 4 weeks.

2. Subchronic toxicity testing

Species:	2 or more.
Exposure time:	For exposure to man of up to 30 days, minimum of 3 months or 1/10th of life span of exposed animals, e.g. 3 months for rats.

3. Chronic toxicity testing

Species: 2, selected on the basis of pharmacokinetics, pharmacodynamics, previous toxicology testing and comparison with human pharmacology.

Exposure time: For exposure to man exceeding 30 days, from 6 months up to full life span in exceptional cases.

4. Combined test, chronic toxicity/carcinogenicity

Difficulty: Achieving optimum condition for both types of experiment simultaneously. Therefore, great care must be taken with experimental design, in particular when deciding number of animals. Further details of carcinogenicity testing, see carcinogenic potential.

Species: 2.

Exposure time: Greater part of life span, mice 18, rats 24 months.

Fetal toxicity

1. Fetal toxicity and teratogenicity testing

Requirement: When drug to be used by women of childbearing potential.

Species: At least 2.
1 for limited test on suspected or known teratogens to determine teratogenic potency.

Dose levels: Preferably 3.

Control groups: Positive control or references from other positive tests where appropriate.

Number of animals: Sufficient number of animals for satisfactory statistical analysis of the data.

Special remarks: A limited test should be carried out on suspected or known teratogens to determine teratogenic potency. One sensitive species will normally be satisfactory.

2. Test for effects on late pregnancy, parturition and lactation

Requirement: When drug likely to be used by women during the later part of pregnancy and/or during the lactation period.

Species: Preferably 2.

Dose levels: At least 3.

Administration period: During last third of pregnancy up to parturition, administration to dams should continue throughout lactation period. Administration to commence on day 12 of pregnancy for mice, on day 15 for rats and on day 18 for rabbits.

Fertility studies

Scope of study: To elucidate any influence of the drug on fertility, general reproductve ability of M and F, and F reproductive cycle. Therefore whole cycle of oogenesis and spermatogenesis must be covered by treatment.

Requirement:	Drugs which might conceivably pose a risk of impaired reproductive function, and when effects on reproductive organs may be suspected, from results obtained in other investigations.
Species:	Normally rats. M at least 6 weeks old at beginning of experiment, F sexually mature.
Administration period:	M for at least 60 days before mating, F for 14 days before mating and during first week of pregnancy.
Experimental procedure:	Studies in which treatment is restricted to M or F may be necessary, in order to determine whether any effects on reproductive capacity relate to one or both sexes.
Methods:	Under development, therefore above guidelines merely one of several possible approaches.
Variables:	Effects on gonadal function, estrus cycle, mating behavior, conception and early stages of gestation.

Carcinogenic potential

Requirement:	When drug is likely to be administered regularly over a substantial period of life, continuously for 6 months or intermittently so that the total exposure is similar. When drug or its metabolites have a chemical structure that suggests a carcinogenic potential. When drug has a mode of action that suggests a risk of carcinogenic potential (e.g. effect on DNA metabolism). When drug belongs to a group of substances members of which have produced positive carcinogenicity test results or have been found to be carcinogenic in epidemiological studies. When its pattern of toxicity or long term retention, including metabolites, suggests a risk (e.g. effect on bone marrow, endocrine glands, spermatogenesis, oogenesis, tumor growth). When drug is found to be positive in mutagenicity tests or short term carcinogenicity tests.
Basis for evaluation:	Chemical structure and mode of action compared to known chemical carcinogens. Results of other toxicity tests, especially teratogenicity and mutagenicity tests as well as chronic toxicity studies in animals.
Species:	Usually 2.
Special remark:	Adequate explanation must be given where carcinogenicity tests are omitted despite fulfilment of one of the above requirements.

Mutagenic potential

Requirement:	All new substances, excipients and other ingredients. Regulatory requirements will vary according to prevailing state of scientific knowledge.

Experimental procedure:	Must cover both gene and chromosome damage.
Methods:	Under development, therefore difficult to issue rigid guidelines. A small number of well-established in vitro and in vivo tests should be applied in combination.

Drugs intended for local application or inhalation

General requirement:	Data on absorption and systemic effects, irritant effects on tissues.

Special investigations

General requirement: Certain drugs require special studies, e.g. of sensitizing properties, influence on immune function, nephrotoxicity (e.g. cephalosporins and non-steroidal anti-inflammatory agents), ototoxicity (e.g. certain antibiotics).

Combination products

General requirement: Toxicological profile of the combination as well as individual components.

Australia

Document reviewed:

AUSTRALIA: Australian Department of Health: NDF 5. Guidelines for Preparation and Presentation of Applications for Investigational Drugs and Drug Products. Draft, August 13, 1987.

Address of Regulatory Agency:

The Secretary, Commonwealth Department of Community Services and Health, P.O. Box 100, Woden, A.C.T., 2606, Australia.

Summary of Toxicological Guidelines:

Acute toxicity

Species:	At least 2 mammalian of known strain (e.g. rodents, such as mouse, rat, hamster). If substantial differences are observed between species, additional species should be studied.
Sex:	Equal numbers of M and F.
Route:	In general 2, including those proposed for clinical use, and at least one ensuring full access of unaltered drug into circulation.
Dose levels:	No exact number is given. Number of dose levels should ensure that full spectrum of toxicity is revealed. In rodents an estimate of the approximate lethality and the dose-effect relationship should be obtained.
Determination of LD50:	A formal estimate of the LD50 is not required.
Observation period:	Adequate to reveal tissue or organ damage or recovery, usually 14 days but not less than 10 days, but without exposing animals to prolonged suffering. If overt signs of toxicity persist, or delayed deaths occur, observation should be continued for a longer period.

Repeated dose toxicity

Species:	At least 2, including a non-rodent, other than rabbit. Pigmented animals to be used with drugs that accumulate in melanin-containing tissues.
Sex:	Depending on expected clinical use, usually M and F.
Route:	As proposed for use in man. When p.o., evidence of absorption should be provided. Oral administration may be substituted for parenteral administration, when metabolic patterns after administration by each route are comparable. When drug is incorporated into diet or drinking water, stability and intake should be monitored.
Dose levels:	At least 3. Highest dose should cause toxic effects. Intermediate dose level(s) for determination of dose-response rela-

Australia

	tionship. Lowest dose should produce appropriate pharmacological or «therapeutic» effects.
Number of animals:	No exact number is given. Size of treatment group should be such that: a) all toxicologically important effects of treatment are revealed, b) animals may be sacrificed at intervals before end of study without interfering with final statistical analysis, c) some animals may be retained at conclusion of administration period to allow evaluation of reversibility of toxic effects.
Duration:	Duration to depend on proposed duration of treatment in humans:

– 1 or several doses in 1 day	2 weeks
– a few days in humans	4 weeks in animals
– up to 1 month in humans	12 weeks in animals
– over 1 month in humans	26 weeks or longer in animals

Reproduction studies

General remarks

Studies are divided into 3 segments: *1) studies of fertility and general reproductive performance, 2) teratogenic* and *3) peri- and postnatal studies.*

No teratology studies will be required in Phase I studies provided that women of child-bearing potential are excluded. Where drug is to be given to F patients of child-bearing potential during the trial, teratogenic studies should have been completed before Phase II clinical trials. Studies on all 3 segments should have been completed before Phase III clinical trials are commenced.

Species:	For 1) and 3): at least 1 mammal.
	For 2) 2 mammals, one a non-rodent (rabbit acceptable).
	Where metabolism of drug in a particular species is known to be similar to that in humans, it is desirable to include this species. It is also desirable that one of the species is same as in long-term toxicity studies.
	Species and strains of animals selected for reproductive studies should neither have a high incidence of spontaneous malformations nor should they be resistant to known teratogens.
Dose levels:	At least 3.
	Maximum dose should be maximum tolerated dose which does not cause significant anorexia, sedation or other adverse effects in the dams; it should produce minimal toxicity, such as relatively decreased body-weight gain. The maximum tolerated dose may not be the same for all 3 study segments and it should be investigated accordingly.
	Intermediate dose should be midway between high and low dose.

Australia

	Minimum dose should be close to pharmacologically active or therapeutically effective dose in the selected species. Preferably, it should produce concentration of drug in blood at least equal to those which occur in man with the proposed clinical dose, if these have already been determined.
	If toxicity data are not available for the species selected, preliminary studies should be conducted and reported in which various dosage levels are administered to the animals and in which the dose that produces maternal toxicity is determined. Only a few animals are required for preliminary studies.
Control groups:	Appropriate control groups should be included.
Route:	Similar to proposed clinical route.
	When p.o., drug should be administered by gavage or in capsules depending on species. When long-term administration is involved, incorporation of drug into food or water may be necessary.
	Quantity of drug absorbed from the proposed site of administration should be known from pharmacokinetic studies.
	I.p. not recommended.
	S.c. should be avoided and substituted by other parenteral routes that provide a greater degree of certainty as to the actual absorption of the drug.

1) Studies of fertility and general reproductive performance

Species:	At least one.
Sex:	M and F.
Number of animals:	If rodents are used, at least 24 M and 24 F per dose.
Route:	Orally or parenterally.
Period of administration:	Daily over at least the period of maturation of the gametes in each sex before mating.
Dose levels:	Where no adverse effect on reproductive performance is produced, evidence should be provided that highest dose was close to a dose which caused toxic effects in the adult animal.
Experimental procedure:	Dosed animals may be mated with dosed partners, but in the event of positive findings of an adverse reproductive effect the study should be repeated using dosed animals mated with undosed partners. Treatment of F should be continued until the young are weaned.
	Some of the F should be killed before parturition and the remainder should be allowed to litter normally.
Variables:	When F are killed: examination of uterus for live, dead and malformed embryos. Effects on duration of pregnancy, malformations and development of the young. Late effects of drug in progeny: growth, development, auditory, visual and behavioral function and reproductive capacity.

Australia

Observation period:	In certain circumstances the young should be observed up to weaning or sexual maturity.

2) Teratogenic studies

Number of animals:	Rodents: at least 20 pregnant F per dose group. Non-rodents: at least 12 pregnant F per dose group.
Period of administration:	Throughout period of organogenesis.
Observation period:	Mother: throughout treatment.
Experimental procedure:	Fetuses should be obtained by Caesarean section shortly before the expected time of parturition.
Variables:	Uterus of mother should be examined for total number of implantations and resorptions, the placentae for anomalies and ovaries for number of corpora lutea. Fetuses should be weighed, measured, classified as live or dead and examined for external malformations. A proportion of the externally malformed and apparently normal fetuses should be dissected and examined for anomalies of internal organs and the remainder for skeletal anomalies.

3) Peri- and postnatal studies

Number of animals:	Rodents: at least 12 pregnant F per dose level.
Period of administration:	To pregnant F throughout final third of gestation and until weaning.
Experimental procedure:	F should be allowed to litter normally and the young observed up to weaning or sexual maturity.
Variables:	Possibility of allowing some of the progeny to live and reach maturity should be considered, so that their reproductive capacity and other effects of the drug, such as alterations of behavioral, learning, visual and auditory functions, may be investigated.

Carcinogenicity

Requirements:	Drugs which – are considered to be closely related chemically or pharmacologically to known or suspected carcinogens – affect mitosis – are likely to be retained in body tissues for a prolonged period – are intended to be given over a prolonged period, especially to young persons – cause concern as a result of findings in mutagenicity studies.
Species:	2. Selection should be made on the basis of metabolic and

Australia

pharmacokinetic similarity to humans. Species and strain susceptibility to a particular carcinogen or class of carcinogens must be considered. Species and strains with a high or variable incidence of spontaneous tumor formation should be avoided.

Sex: M and F.

Duration of study: Rat: at least 24 months. Mouse and hamster: at least 18 months. Where survival rate is high there may be advantages in extending these times. When cumulative mortality is such that prolongation of study is no longer statistically justified, study should be terminated prematurely.

Number of animals: At least 50 of each sex per group.

Control groups: 2, 50 animals of each sex per group.

Dose levels: At least 3.

Highest dose should be maximum tolerated dose as predicted from shorter studies. Maximum tolerated dose = highest dose which does not produce signs of toxicity or pathologic lesions which would be expected to shorten the animal's natural life span. Intermediate dose should be midway between high and low dose.

Low dose should permit animals to survive in good health for their natural life span or until tumors develop. It should be near the pharmacologically or therapeutically effective dose. If signs of toxicity appear during the course of the study, appropriate action should be taken to ensure adequate survival of adequate numbers of animals. Depending on the objectives of the study, dose may be lowered, discontinued or the dosage regimen changed.

Administration: Normally daily.

Route: As proposed for use in man. When p.o., decision whether by gavage or in diet or drinking water must be made. When given in food or water, stability data required.- Parenteral administration on a frequent chronic basis may cause local pathology unrelated to carcinogenicity *per se* of drug. In this case, weekly or less frequent injections throughout study may be considered.- When metabolic patterns appear to be independent of route, oral administration may be an adequate substitute for parenteral administration.

Mutagenicity

Requirements: All drugs which
– are to be used over a period of years, particulary by children and young adults, used for general prophylaxis or which come into contact with sperm at a high concentration;
– are considered to be closely related chemically, pharmacol-

ogically or biochemically to known or suspected mutagens;
– are known to depress bone marrow at tolerated dose levels;
– are known to be teratogenic at maximum tolerated dose;
– are known to inhibit gametogenesis in animals or to reduce fertility in reproductive studies;
– are known to produce carcinogenic effects;
– are unrelated to known pharmacological agents.

Species / cells: Microorganisms, mammalian cells in culture, insects, mammals.

Method: Several tests should be used for each drug, since different tests detect different mutational events, e.g. chromosomal and point mutations, sister chromatid exchanges. Selection of tests should be justified by investigator.

Evaluation of results: Positive or negative in vitro results at the prescreening stage are insufficient for valid assessment of drug safety as regards mutagenicity.
Results should be confirmed in whole-animal systems. Evidence which might militate against positive in vitro results should be discussed.

Drugs to be applied to mucosal or dermal surfaces

Such drugs should be studied on the corresponding tissues in animals. Results obtained in one type of tissue are not necessariliy applicable to other tissues. If product is an aerosol, possible accidental inhalation should be considered. Amount and type of testing should be determined according to proposed indications for use and exposure conditions as well as site of application.

Studies should include:
a) Pharmacodynamic studies
b) Pharmacokinetic studies
c) Microbiological studies, if appropriate
d) Acute toxicity studies
e) Repeat dose toxicity studies
f) Local toxicity studies:
Primary irritant potential of drug and/or formulation to be used clinically, both acute and cumulative, should be determined in appropriate species. Where formulation is intended for dermal application it should be tested on both intact and abraded skin. Studies of potential for phototoxicity, photosensitivity and dermal sensitization should be considered.
g) Mutagenicity studies
h) Carcinogenicity studies. Skin carcinogenicity studies may be required.

Drugs for inhalation other than volatile anaesthetics

Choice of appropriate test procedures should be made according to physical and chemical properties and proposed clinical use of product. Drug(s) should be evaluated in the form of proposed final formulation, with particle size and densitiy being controlled and kept constant. Propellant system used in studies should be that proposed for the final product. If a novel propellant system is used, it should be investigated to the same standard as the active substance.

Studies should include: see above, except c) and f)

Volatile anaesthetics for inhalation

Studies should include: see above, except c) and f)

Intravenous infusion fluids and plastic or plastic lined containers for such fluids

Requirements for toxicity testing depend on ingredients of fluids and, in some cases, on type of storage container. Separate tests for:
- Amino acids, fats, sugars, alcohols and electrolytes.
- Artificial blood products.
- Plastic containers.

Austria

Document reviewed:

AUSTRIA: Bundesgesetzblatt für die Republik Oesterreich, 82. Verordnung: Arzneispezialitätenverordnung – ASpV, February 28, 1985.

Addresses of Regulatory Agencies:

– Bundeskanzleramt, Ballhausplatz 2, A-1014 Wien.
– Bundesanstalt für experimentell-pharmakologische und balneologische Untersuchungen, Währingerstrasse 13 a, A-1090 Wien.

Summary of Toxicological Guidelines:

Acute toxicity

Species:	More than one mammal.
Route:	More than one, one route same as or similar to that proposed for use in man, one to ensure absorption of substance.
Observation period:	2 weeks after administration.
Variables:	Toxic signs.

Repeated dose toxicity

Species:	More than one mammal, one a non-rodent.
Sex:	M and F.
Route:	Same as or similar to that proposed for use in man.
Duration:	According to maximum intended therapeutic duration of drug.
Dose levels:	3, one to cause toxic signs, one of the order of magnitude of that proposed for clinical use.
Control group:	At least one.
Number of animals:	Adequate number for each group.
Variables:	Toxic signs and any observation on live, dead and sacrificed animals.
Special remarks:	The evaluation of the data should address the question of possible indications of carcinogenic or immunomodulating effect.

Reproduction studies

General remarks

Purpose: To elucidate effect on reproduction, i.e. mating behavior and fertility, loss of embryos and fetuses or late effect on offspring. Toxic effects during preimplantation or implantation period, or on embryo or fetus. Effects on physiology of the dam, on intrauterine growth and development and placenta, interference with parturition. Effects on postnatal development, e.g. on nursing behavior of offspring.

Embryotoxicity

Species:	2 mammalian, one a non-rodent.
Period of administration:	During organogenesis.
Dose levels:	3, one to cause slight toxic signs on dam, one of the order of magnitude of that proposed for clinical use.
Number of animals:	Adequate number for each group.
Control groups:	At least one.
Experimental procedure:	Fetuses removed by Caesarean section.

Reproduction studies

Species:	At least one mammal.
Sex:	Fertile M and F.
Duration:	At least two generations.
Dose levels:	See embryotoxicity.
Number of animals:	See embryotoxicity.
Control groups:	See embryotoxicity.
Experimental procedure:	Fetuses removed by Caesarean section and spontaneous delivery.

Carcinogenicity

Requirement:	All drugs (including excipients and contaminants) – proposed to be administered over significant fraction of life span – that are chemically related to known carcinogens – that have revealed in previous toxicity tests effects suggesting carcinogenic potential – that have revealed in genotoxicity tests and other short-term tests evidence of carcinogenic properties
Species:	More than one mammal (results of repeated-dose toxicity tests may be used if requirements below are met).
Sex:	M and F.
Number of animals:	Adequate number for each group.
Duration:	Adequate duration.
Control groups:	At least one.

Mutagenicity

General remarks

Several well established in vitro and in vivo tests should be applied in combination according to chemical structure and physico-chemical properties of drug.

Aim of these tests: Examination of genome-, gene- and chromosome mutations, metabolism of drug in mammalian organism in vitro and in vivo, and positive and negative controls using substances with known effects. No specific tests are recommended.

Local effects
Local effects of drugs not intended for oral application should be tested.

Intravenous application
Data are required on venous, paravenous, and intraarterial tolerance to drugs intended for intravenous application .

External application
Sensitizing properties of drugs to be used externally or in the eyes should be tested.
Drugs to be used systemically should be tested for their sensitizing properties, when:
– the preparation procedure
– the composition
– the pharmacokinetic properties of the drug or its components
– the chemical similarity of the components to known sensitizing substances
imply possibility of sensitizing effects.

Inhalation toxicity
Tests on inhalation toxicity are required for drugs intended for inhalation. No specific tests are recommended.

Radioactivity
The pre-clinical data for drugs intended to be used in conjunction with radioactive drugs should include the following information:
– biological distribution of the radioactive material when administered by a specific route, including quantitative data on uptake (accumulation) in various organs
– excretion of radioactive drugs and determination of biological half-life
– the absorbed fraction of the radiation dose per unit of administered activity in particular in the target organ, the hemopoietic organs, the reticuloendotelial system, the M and F sex organs and the whole body
– the medium absorbed radioactive dose in the target organ after single administration (in this experiment the administered dose must take into account organ and body weight)
– the mean cumulative absorbed radiation dose in the target organ must also be determined if the radioactive drug is given repeatedly
– radiation from radioactive impurities
– toxicological influence of substances emanating from radiolysis.

Belgium

BELGIUM uses the **EEC-Guidelines** and the **«Arrêté Royal»**.

Document reviewed:

BELGIUM: Ministère de la Santé Publique et de la Famille: Arrêté royal concernant les normes et protocoles applicables en matière d'essais de médicaments à usage humain. September 16, 1985 (Published in Moniteur Belge, November 13, 1985).

Address of Regulatory Agency:

Commission des Médicaments, Ministère de la Santé publique et de la Famille, Inspection générale de la Pharmacie, Cité administrative de l'Etat, quartier Ve-'sale, B-1010 Bruxelles.

Note:

The toxicological guidelines, mentioned in the above document are identical to the EEC-Guidelines I, Part 2, Chapter 1, A – E.

Peoples' Republic of Benin

Document rewieved:

PEOPLES' REPUBLIC OF BENIN: Letter from the director of the Ministry of Health, October 13, 1987.

Address of Regulatory Agency:

Direction des Pharmacies au Ministère de la Santé Publique, BP 2048, Cotonou, République Populaire du Bénin.

Note:

Peoples' Republic of Benin has no own specific guidelines. The registration of new drugs is essentially based on the tests and documents of the original manufacturer. If the country of origin of a drug is France, the »AMM« (Autorisation de Mise sur le Marché) should be submitted. If the country of origin is the FRG or Switzerland, the current marketing licence should be submitted.

Brasil

Document reviewed:

BRASIL: Conselho Nacional de Saude, Câmara Tecnica de Alimentos, Resolucao Normativa no. 1/78. Diario Oficial, October 17, 1978.

Address of Regulatory Agency:

Secretaria Nacional de Vigilância Sanitaria do Ministerio da Saude, Brasilia – DF – CEP 70058.

Summary of Toxicological Guidelines:

Acute toxicity (less than 24 hours)

Species:	At least 3, one a non-rodent.
Number of animals:	To be reported.
Route:	Route proposed for use in man plus one other.
Dose levels:	To be reported.
Determination of LD50:	LD 50 required. LD5 and LD95 in some cases.
Methods:	To be described.
Variables:	Toxic signs, acute potentiation (in combinations with other drugs).

Subacute Toxicity (12 to 24 weeks)

Species:	At least 2, one a non-rodent.
Number of animals:	To be reported.
Route:	To be reported.
Dose levels:	At least 3
Methods:	To be described.
Variables:	Behavior, weight, food intake, hematology, blood chemistry, hepatic and renal functions, electrolytes, anatomy and histopathology, ophthalmology, ECG, neurology, urinalysis, blood concentration of substance, mortality. New combinations with other drugs.

Chronic toxicity (6 or more months)

Species:	At least 2, one a non-rodent.
Number of animals:	To be reported.
Route:	To be reported.
Dose levels:	At least 3.

Brasil

Methods:	To be described.
Variables:	See subacute toxicity.

Teratogenesis and embryotoxicity

Species:	At least 3, one a non-rodent.
Number of animals:	To be reported.
Route:	To be reported.
Dose levels:	To be reported.
Methods:	To be reported.
Variables:	To be reported.

Special studies

Fertility and reproductive capacity, carcinogenesis, mutagenesis, local irritation, sensitivization, pharmacotechnical studies, compatibility of substances with the vehicle, toxicity of new vehicles, others (to be reported).

Canada

Document rewieved:

CANADA: Bureau of Human Prescription Drugs – Health Protection Branch – Health and Welfare Canada. Preclinical Toxicologic Guidelines. June 1981.

Address of Regulatory Agency:

Bureau of Human Prescription Drugs, Health Protection Branch, Health and Welfare Canada, Tunney's Pasture, Ottawa, Ontario, Canada K1A OL2.

Summary of Toxicological Guidelines:

Acute toxicity

Species:	At least 3 (2 rodents and one non-rodent other than rabbit), including those species used in pharmacologic testing and those likely to be used in long-term and special toxicity studies. Additional species if substantial species differences are observed.
Sex:	M and F unless clinical use of drug precludes its employment in both sexes in man.
Route:	– Parenteral drugs: All parenteral routes to be used clinically (also i.v., even if i.v. is not proposed for clinical use) – Oral drugs: p.o. and a parenteral route (i.v. or i.p.).
Rate of administration:	For i.v. route not less than 0.1 ml/sec.
Dose levels:	3 or more doses other than LD50 and LD100 (rodents). Control test with vehicle alone.
Vehicle control:	That which is proposed for clinical use.
Experimental animals:	Animals should be about the same age and, within each sex, body weight should not vary more than 10 %.
Number of animals:	– Rodents: in final tests at least 10 of each sex per dose. – Non-rodents: small number, sufficient for determination of approximate LD50 or MLD.
Observation period:	At least 10 days or longer, if toxic signs persist or delayed deaths occur.
Determination of LD:	LD50 with confidence limit, minimal lethal dose (MLD) or a tolerance level. When not possible, because of low acute toxicity of drug, tolerance tests may be substituted in rodents and/or non-rodents.
Experimental detail:	When determining LD50 by oral route, animals should be fasted prior to the assay but may have access to a 10 % aqueous solution of glucose. Fasting animals before acute toxicity studies recommended, whatever the route.

Variables:	Signs of toxicity including onset and duration (effects on locomotion, behavior, respiration, circulation, etc.). Time and cause of death, autopsy when delayed deaths occur and in some cases histopathology. Species, sex and age differences. Dose-response curve. Delayed toxicity.

Long-term toxicity

Species:	At least 2, including a non-rodent (other than rabbit).
Sex:	According to expected clinical use of drug, but usually M and F.
Duration:	4 weeks for dose-range studies prior to long-term tests. 4 to 6 weeks, not longer than 3 months for initial toxicity studies (before the drug has been administered to man). Longer studies in species that resembles man metabolically. Final or definitive long-term toxicity studies may last for several years or more. See Table: «Minimal toxicological requirements», p 61.
Administration:	When drug is to be administered to man daily, it should be given to animal 7 days per week. If other regimen used, justification to be supplied.
Route:	Route to be used in clinical studies. When p.o., evidence for absorption should be provided. When drug in diet, stability and intake should be monitored. P.o. instead of parenteral administration possible, if metabolic patterns of both routes shown to be comparable.
Dose levels:	At least 3. Highest to cause toxic effects but allow survival of majority of animals. Lowest should be effective dose for species concerned. One or more intermediate dose levels for determination of dose-response relationships. Vehicle-treated controls and in special cases positive and/or non-treated controls required.
Number of animals:	– Rodents: sufficient to permit periodic laboratory investigations and histopathology and information on reversibility. – Non-rodents: smaller number of animals.
Variables:	Changes in appearance and behavior, neurological effects, body weight, food and water consumption; hematology, clinical chemistry, urinalysis, occult fecal blood and liver and kidney function tests where applicable. Eye examination of all non-rodents. Neurotoxicity, functional and structural abnormalities of the special sense organs where applicable. Cardiovascular as well as other physiological and pharmacological manifestations should be monitored where practicable. All major organs should be weighed and examined for gross pathological changes. Histopathology in high-dose and control groups. Lower doses also, if gross and microscopic

changes found at high dose. Hematology, clinical chemistry and urinalysis of all recovery animals.

Local response of tissue at site of administration. Irritation studies and compatibility with blood for parenterally administered drugs. In special cases electron microscopy, fluorescent antibodies, histochemical and autoradiographic procedures may be required.

Reproductive studies
General remarks

Route:	Should be similar to the proposed clinical route. Topical drugs should be administered topically. I.p. administration not recommended, s.c. should be avoided.
Dose levels:	3, maximum dose should be the maximum tolerated dose, or should produce only minimal toxicity. Lower dose should be close to effective dose in the selected species, or to proposed therapeutic dose. Intermediate dose should be midway between high and low dose. A control group to which the vehicle alone is administered should always be included. In special cases control group, which receives handling, but neither vehicle nor drug.
Age:	Where possible, animals used in experimental and control groups within a study should always be of comparable age.
Number of animals:	For fertility studies: at least 30 F and 15 M per group. For teratogenicity and peri- and postnatal studies: at least 20 pregnant F for rodents and 15 pregnant F for non-rodents.
Animal husbandry:	Animal maintenance and care should meet high standards, and all environmental factors should be carefully controlled and recorded.

a) Study of fertility and general reproductive performance (Segment I)

Species:	At least one, rat (or mouse)
Sex:	M and F.
Age:	M: at least 40 days before drug administration begins. F: at least sexually mature.
Administration:	M: 80 days prior to mating. F: 14 days before exposure to M, continued daily until sacrifice or until weaning.
Number of animals:	As a minimum 15 M should be mated with 30 F.
Experimental detail:	M from subacute or chronic drug toxicity studies may be used. These pretreated M can be mated with either treated or non-treated F.
Method:	– 50 % of F sacrificed on day 13 of pregnancy. – 50 % of F: spontaneous delivery.

Variables:	– Hysterectomy: examination of uterus, number and distribution of embryos in each uterine horn, implantations and resorptions. – Spontaneous delivery: duration of gestation, litter size, still born and live born, gross anomalies. Dead pups: skeletal anomalies. Birth weight of pups and weight on day 4 and 21, effort to determine cause of any observed adverse effects. In certain circumstances the young should be allowed to live and reach maturity for studies of late effects of the drug (auditory, visual and behavioral function and reproductive capacity).

b) Teratological study (Segment II)

Species:	At least 2, normally mouse, rat and rabbit.
Administration:	Throughout period of organ formation (mouse and rat 6th to 15th day, rabbit 6th to 18th day of pregnancy).
Method:	Hysterectomy 1 or 2 days prior to parturition.
Variables:	Number of fetuses, their placement in the uterine horn, correlation with number of corpora lutea, live and dead fetuses, early and late resorptions. Fetuses should be weighed and examined for external anomalies and internal defects. Division of fetuses at random into 2 groups for different kinds of examination, e.g. 1/3 for dissection, 2/3 for bone staining.

c) Perinatal and postnatal study (Segment III)

Administration:	Final one-third of gestation throughout lactation to weaning.
Observation period:	Some of the offspring until maturity for investigation of their reproductive capacity and late effects of the drug (behavioral, learning, visual and auditory functions).
Special Methods:	Cross-fostering of some litters between control and high-dose dams.
Variables:	Labor, delivery, duration of gestation, litter size, pup weight.

Carcinogenicity

Requirement:	Before administration to man: when chemical and biological properties of drug resemble those of a known carcinogen, when metabolites with similar properties are formed from both the drug and a known carcinogen; when drug damages rapidly growing tissues in relatively short experiments; or when it affects mitosis. Exception: no carcinogenicity study necessary for antineoplastic drugs used in terminally ill patients.
Species:	2, usually rat, mouse or hamster. In special cases dog, primate, or other. Species with known susceptibility to particular carcinogen. Inbred strain that is known to respond to

particular test compound for study of basic mechanism in carcinogenesis. Animals with heterogeneous genetic constitution for determination of potential carcinogenicity of a hitherto untested compound. Metabolic pathways in man and in the animal species must be considered. SPF animals recommended. Spontaneous tumor incidence, sensitivity to tumor induction, availability, genetic stability, etc. of the species and strain selected should be known.

Sex: M and F, unless drug is to be restricted to one sex in man.

Age: Not older than 6 weeks, and if possible weanlings at the start of the study. Sometimes, in utero exposures.

Duration: Greater part of animal's life span (rats, mice and hamsters: at least 24 months).

Route: Same as proposed for use in man.
– When p.o., decision whether by gavage or in diet or drinking water (stability studies necessary).
– When parenteral: this route on a chronic basis in animals may cause pathology unrelated to the carcinogenicity *per se* of drug. Consideration of less frequent injections.
– When metabolic patterns appear to be independent of route, p.o. administration may be an adequate substitute for parenteral administration.
– When appropriate tissue concentrations of parent drug and/or metabolite(s) are not attained in animals by route to be used clinically another route that produces such concentrations should be sought.

Dose levels: At least 3. Highest should be the maximum tolerated dose (M.T.D.) as predicted from 3 months studies; lowest should permit the animals to survive in good health for their natural life span or until tumors develop, dose should be near the effective dose for that species. Third dose should be around midway between high and low dosage levels. Additional control groups, most commonly vehicle-treated, may be necessary. Positive controls only when new chemical is structurally similar to known carcinogen. Colony controls should be kept.

Number of animals: At least 50 animals per sex and per treatment. 2 control groups, each with 50 animals per sex, are recommended. Sometimes additional control groups necessary, e.g. vehicle control or exposure to nitrogen and oxygen in studies with inhalation anesthetics.

Animal husbandry: Environmental conditions and general care of animals must be under control. Diets free of common carcinogens. Semisynthetic diets to be considered.

Observations: Frequent and complete animal surveillance. Viability check of every animal once in the morning and once in the after-

Canada

Variables:	noon 7 days per week. Time of onset, location, size and growth characteristics of any unusual tissue masses, food and water consumption, animal weights, autopsy on all animals, histopathology on all organs and tissues of high dose and control groups and organs and tissues showing gross changes in animals of other groups. Organs showing increased tumor incidence in high dose group must also be examined in other groups. All tissues from all animals should be stored for 10 years.

Mutagenicity

Requirements:	All drugs and/or metabolite(s) – that are chemically, biochemically or pharmacologically related to known mutagens – that produce certain biological effects (e.g. depression of gametogenesis, fertility, immunity or hematopoiesis at maximum tolerated doses) – that are often used over a period of years, particularly in children and young adults – that come in contact with sperms.
Species:	Microorganisms, cultures of mammalian cells, insects and mammals.
Methods:	No standard battery of tests can be recommended, only that a battery of several tests should be used: tests that detect chromosomal and point mutations and sister chromatid exchanges should be used for each drug. Some tests can be run concomitantly with long-term toxicity and reproductive tests (e.g. micronucleus and sperm morphology test).

Topical studies

1. Primary irritation potential

Species:	Rabbit and guinea pig. When other species are used, standard irritants with related chemical and physical properties and with known irritancy in rabbits and guinea pigs should be tested with the unknown formulation to ascertain relative reactivity of the species selected.
Test procedure:	Depending on chemical structure(s) of the various compound(s) of the formulation. Large variety of procedures described in current literature. No specific battery of tests recommended.

1.1. Acute primary irritation of the skin

Species:	Rabbit and/or guinea pig.
Number of animals:	At least 6.

Test procedure:	Modifications of Draize method are considered adequate. Rabbit – and/or guinea pig test, depending on type of material to be tested.
Exposure time:	Standard, 24-hour, occlusive patch test and 4-hour, semi-occlusive patch test not always adequate. Conditions of clinical use or special properties of material could require shorter or longer exposures. A variable time of exposure which produces a definite, irritant end-point may be preferable.
Variables:	Erythema, edema or more severe reactions such as eschar formation and necrosis. Stinging, burning sensation and itching potential in man are not usually predictable from animal studies.

1.2. Cumulative irritation

Exposure time:	Repeated applications to animal skin for 7 to 21 days.
Variables:	Same as in 1.1.

1.3. Phototoxicity (due to light-activated chemical)

Species:	Hairless mice, rabbits, swine and guinea pigs.
Number of animals:	Not less than 6 per group.
U.V. light:	Usually between 320 and 450 nm. Intervals between drug administration and U.V. radiation carefully controlled and kept constant.

2. Photosensitivity potential (photoallergy)

Species:	Guinea pig.
Number of animals:	Generally 10 to 25 per group.
Test procedure:	Basically: induction period in which product is applied to shaved skin of animals and treated area is later exposed to U.V. radiation. This procedure is repeated daily for varying periods of time.
Administration period:	Challenge dose administered about 2 weeks after induction period and consists of an application of the product to 2 previously untreated areas of skin and exposing one of these areas to U.V. radiation, while other area is kept covered and receives no radiation.

3. Allergic contact dermatitis potential

Species:	Guinea pig. Genetic factors are important: outbred strains for the detection of strong sensitizers, inbred strains for weak sensitizers recommended. No pregnant animals, as pregnancy decreases cutaneous expression of sensitization.
Age:	1 to 3-months-old.
Number of animals:	10 to 20 per group. Untreated control animals should also be challenged.

Canada

Induction:	Intradermal or topical on back or nuchal area. 10 doses, 2 to 3 days' interval.
Dose:	Challenge dose usually lower concentration than induction dose, administered about 2 weeks after last induction dose. Dose can be manipulated by varying concentration, number of exposures, area involved and volume administered.
Adjuvants:	For enhancement of sensitization. Should be given together with test formulation or separately near site of administration, together with or a few days after but not before administration of allergen.
Observation:	Reaction is read at 24 hrs and subsequently if necessary.
Note:	For weak sensitizers the guinea pig maximization test or the open epicutaneous test may be used.

4. Effects on skin pigmentation

Species:	Guinea pig.
Test procedure:	Techniques for determining leukoderma now available, they should be conducted when appropriate.

5. Effects on flora

When topical agents are to be applied to a major portion of skin or mucosal surface, possible microbial modifications should be evaluated.

6. Effect on healing

When a formulation is intended for application to wounds, burns or traumatized skin, it is necessary to ascertain whether it accelerates or delays healing.

7. Substantivity (retention on or in skin)

Minimal skin penetrants with high substantivity might produce adverse systemic effects owing to their prolonged cutaneous penetration.

8. Prolonged topical toxicity on skin or mucous membranes

Species:	Rabbit, miniature pig, rat and monkey.
Application period:	Daily to shaved skin during period of time that varies according to proposed duration of clinical use.
Dose levels:	3 plus control group.
Test procedure:	If percutaneous absorption studies show that active ingredient(s) and/or vehicle are not absorbed, then only local effects need be studied. If absorption has been shown, oral and parenteral LD50 required. If absorption is considerable, possibility of conducting long-term studies by oral or parenteral routes also should be considered.

9. Eye irritation

Species:	Rabbit and/or monkey.
Number of animals:	At least 6 per treatment group.

Canada

Application period:	For short-term clinical use: a) for single application in man, 5-day ocular irritation tests, b) for therapeutic trials lasting up to a few weeks, a 21-day ocular irritation test. For long-term clinical use: 6-months test.
Dosage regimen:	Similar to that proposed clinically.

Systemic studies

Species:	Rabbit (for topical LD50), rat, miniature pig or monkey.
Sex:	M and F.
Number of animals:	At least 5 per sex and concentration.
Concentrations of product:	3 or more.
Exposure time:	24 hrs.
Determination of LD50:	Approximate LD50 if possible.
Test procedure:	Various methods, including chemical analyses, bioassays and use of radioactive compounds.

Inhalation studies

Test procedure:	Either masks or endotracheal administration for acute studies, exposure chambers for long-term studies.
Selection of species:	Additional consideration should be given to different anatomic and physiological characteristics of respiratory systems in different species. (Rabbits, dogs and monkeys can adapt to mouth breathing, when their nasal passages are blocked, mice and rats cannot).

Canada

Tables of minimal toxicological requirements

Category	Expected Duration of Therapy	Phase	Duration of Human Trial	Acute Toxicity	Long-term Toxicity	R.St.	M.G.	C.G.
A. Oral or parenteral drugs	Up to 1 week	Clinical pharmacol.	up to 1 week	3 or more species, oral and parenteral	2 species 4-6 weeks			(+)
		Therap. trial	1 week		2 species* 8 weeks	(+)		(+)
		N.D.S.	---		2 species 4-6 mos.**	(+)	(+)	(+)
	up to 1 month	Clinical pharmacol.	up to 1 week	as above	2 species 4-6 weeks			(+)
		Therap. trial	1 to 4 weeks		2 species* 12 weeks	(+)	(+)	
		N.D.S.	---		2 species* R & non-R: 18 mos**	+	(+)	(+)
A 1. Single ingredient	1 month to 1 year	Clinical pharmacol.	up to 1 week	as above	2 species 4-6 weeks			(+)
			1 to 4 weeks		2 species* 12 weeks			
		Therap. trial	up to 1 month		2 species* 12 weeks			
			more than 1 month		2 species* R:12-18mos non-R:12mos	(+)		(+)
		N.D.S.	---		2 species* R & non-R:(+) 18mos**	(+)	(+)	(+)
A 1. Single ingredient	1 year or more	Clinical pharmacol.	up to 1 week	as above	2 species 4-6 weeks			(+)
			up to 4 weeks		2 species* 12 weeks			
		Therap. trial	1 month to 1 year		2 species* R & non-R:(+) 12-18mos	(+)	(+)	(+)
		N.D.S.	---		2 species* R & non-R: + 18mos**	(+)	(+)	(+)

R.St. = Reproductive Studies; M.G. = Mutagenesis; C.G. = Carcinogenesis

* Metabolic studies have been done, species selected are as similar to man as possible.

** Duration of studies should be extended according to existing toxicity data, nature of drug, proposed clinical use and indications. 18-months, chronic toxicity studies in rodents will not be considered as substitutes for carcinogenicity studies, which should last at least 24 months in these species.

(+) Signifies that studies may or may not be required according to nature of drug, similarity with known mutagens and/or carcinogens, retention within the organism, toxicity data to date and proposed clinical use.

R = Rodent; non-R = non-rodent.

Canada

Category	Expected Duration of Therapy	Phase	Duration of Human Trial	Acute Toxicity	Long-term Toxicity	R.St.	M.G.	C.G.
A. Oral	A few days	Clinical pharmac.	up to 1 week	2 species, oral	2 species 4-6 weeks			(+)
or parenteral	to more than	Therap. trial	1 week to more than 1 year	and	2 apecies 3 months (a) (b)	(+)	(+)	(+)
drugs	1 year	N.D.S.	---	parenteral		+	(+)	(+)
A 2. Multiple ingredients								

R.St. = Reproductive Studies; M.G. = Mutagenesis; C.G. = Carcinogenesis
(a) Adequate toxicity data should be available for the individual drugs.
(b) If the individual drugs interact to significantly modify pharmacological and/or toxicological activity, long-term toxicity studies should be conducted for 1 year in the non-rodent and for at least 18 months in the rodent.

Category	Expected Duration of Therapy	Phase	Duration of Human Trial	Minimal Studies to be Conducted before Initiating trials in corresponding Phase
B. Topical drugs B 1. Dermal	Single or short-term application up to a few weeks	a) Clin. pharm.	Single application	Acute toxicity by topical route. Acute primary irritation potential. 1 or 2 species as appropriate.
		b) Therap. trial	a few weeks	Cumulative irritation potential. Phototoxicity and photoallergy if applicable. Sensitization potential. Oral LD 50. Percutaneous absorption.
		c) N.D.S.	---	Special studies as appropriate. Long-term studies in 2 species in accordance with proposed duration of use.
	Unlimited application	d) Clin. pharm.	Single application	As for B. B 1.a
		e) Therap. trial	short-term (a few wks)	As for B. B 1.b
			long-term (a few mos)	Prolonged topical toxicity extended according to duration of clinical use. Special studies as appropriate.
		f) N.D.S.	---	Special studies as appropriate. Longterm studies in 2 species in accordance with proposed duration of use.* Skin carcinogenicity studies if indicated. Other special studies as appropriate.

Canada

* In the event of significant absorption, regular long-term toxicity studies should be conducted using the topical route or, if the metabolic profile is not affected by the route of administration, using the oral or parenteral routes. Duration and dosage determined by proposed clinical use. Species as indicated in text for each type of study.

Category	Expected Duration of Therapy	Phase	Duration of Human Trial	Minimal Studies to be Conducted before Initiating Trials in Corresponding Phase
B. Topical drugs B 2. Ophthalmic	Single or short-term application for a few weeks to 2 months	a) Clin. pharm.	Single application	5-day irritation test. 1 or 2 species as appropriate (rabbit and/or monkey).
		b) Therap. trial	a few weeks	21-day irritation test. Local toxicity. Clinical and histopathologic examination where appropriate. Systemic toxicity where necessary. 2 species.
		c) N.D.S.	---	Long-term topical and, if absorbed, general toxicity studies in 2 species; duration in accordance to length of proposed clinical use.
	unlimited application	d) Clin. pharm.	Single application	As for B. B2.a
		e) Therap. trial	a few weeks	As for B. B2.b
			a few months	Long-term topical and, if absorbed, general toxicity studies in 2 species; duration in accordance to length of proposed clinical use.
		f) N.D.S.	---	Long-term topical and, if absorbed, general toxicity studies in 2 species; duration in accordance to length of proposed clinical use.

Canada

Category	Expected Duration of Therapy	Phase	Duration of Human Trial	Minimal Studies to be Conducted before Initiating Trials in Corresponding Phase
B. Topical drugs B 3. Rectal	---	---	---	**Rectal preparation intended to produce systemic effects should be investigated for: 1) systemic toxicity,** species and duration of studies as indicated for oral and parenteral drugs; route should be proposed clinical route if possible (oral or parenteral acceptable if metabolic patterns are not affected by route of administration). 2) **local toxicity**, 2 species; duration in accordance with proposed duration of use. **Rectal preparations intended to produce only local effects should be investigated for local toxicity,** 2 species; duration of studies in accordance with proposed duration of use. Lack of absorption should be adequately demonstrated.
B 4. **Vaginal**	---	---	---	**Vaginal preparations intended to produce local effects should be investigated for local toxicity.** Lack of absorption should be adequately demonstrated. Reproductive and other special studies may be required depending on the proposed clinical use.

Category	Expected Duration of Therapy	Phase	Duration of Human Trial	Acute Toxicity	Long-term Toxicity	R.St.	M.G.	C.G.
C. Inhalation drugs C 1. General anaesthetics	Single administration for various exposure times	Clin. pharm.	Single administration (Short exposure)	4 or more species 3 or more exposure times	3 or more species 2 or more exposure times 3 or more concentrations (if possible) 2-4 weeks			
		Therap. trial	Single administration (long exposures)	as above	as above, except, that duration extended to 4 weeks adequate exposure times (+)			
		N.D.S.	---	as above	3 or more species 4-6 months	+	(+)	(+)

64

Canada

C 2. Other inha- lants	Acute, long-term and special studies as indicated for oral and parenteral drugs, as regards duration of studies and number of species. 3 or more durations of exposure and, if possible, concentrations should be used in the acute studies; at least 2 exposure times should be used in the long-term studies; proposed clinical exposure time and a multiple thereof so as to simulate exaggerated use.

R.st. = Reproductive Studies; M.G. = Mutagenesis; C.G. = Carcinogenesis
(+) Signifies that studies may or may not be required according to nature of drug, similarity with known mutagens and/or carcinogens, retention within organism, toxicity data to date and proposed clinical use.

Chile

Note:

CHILE has no rules or guidelines for safety testing of new drugs. Usually the pre-clinical information presented for obtaining the registration of a new product is based on data from other countries or from scientific publications and is evaluated by members of scientific societies and then submitted for consideration by the National Commission on Drugs, an advisory group of the Ministry of Health.

For general and specific provisions for the regulation of pharmaceutical products consult the Law Force Decree No. 725, December 1967 and Decree No. 425 of 1981 (not summarized).

Address of Regulatory Agency:

Departamento de Control Nacional, Instituto de Salud Publica de Chile, Maraton 1000, Santiago-Chile.

Diagnostic products: Not subjected to registrational control.

People's Republic of China

Document reviewed:
PEOPLE'S REPUBLIC OF CHINA: Provisions for New Drug Approval. July 1, 1985.

Address of Regulatory Agency:
Division of Modern Drugs, Bureau of Drug Administration and Policy, Ministry of Public Health, Beijing, People's Republic of China.

Summary of Toxicological Guidelines:
Acute toxicity

Species:	Not indicated.
Route:	Not less than 2, one same as proposed for use in man.
LD50:	Determination of LD50 required, also i.v. LD50, if test drug is water-soluble.
Observation period:	At least 7 days.
Variables:	Gross necropsy and record of all pathological changes when toxic reactions appear. Microscopic examination of tissues showing pathological changes, also of animals which survived for 24 hours or more.

Long-term toxicity test

Scope of study:	To determine toxic reactions of animals to continuous administration of test drug, including initial signs, progressive damage to tissues and their function, and reversibility.
Species:	At least 2, rodent and non-rodent.
Sex:	M and F.
Age:	Rats usually 6 weeks, dogs usually 4-6 months.
Number of animals:	To depend on experimental period. Rodents: 10 of each sex per group if period is less than 90 days. 20 of each sex per group, if period is more than 90 days. Non-rodents (usually dogs): 2 of each sex per group.
Controls:	Equal numbers of animals in control group as in test groups.
Route:	For parenteral use same as proposed for use in man, for oral use preferably via stomach tube.
Dose levels:	Normally 3. For large animals 2. Highest dose should cause toxic reactions or death in some animals (20 %), low dose should be slightly higher than effective dose and observation indicators should cause no toxic effect.
Observation period:	If new drug produces toxic reactions, observation of high-dose group and control group should be continued even after conclusion of administration period.

China

Duration:	To depend on duration of proposed clinical use:

	in man:	in animal:
	– 1-3 days	2 weeks
	– 7 or 30 days	4 or 12 weeks
	– more than 30 days	6 months
	– more than 6 months	Application for phase I clinical trial may be submitted after 3 months if no significant toxic reactions are observed

Variables:	General physical signs, weight, appearance, behavior, routine blood and urine test, liver and kidney function tests, gross and histopathological examinations of important organs, bone marrow examination, blood biochemistry; in large animals: heart rate and ECG.
	For drugs liable to be toxic to eyes or ears, observation indicators for these special toxicities should be added. Influence on acid-base balance and water-salt metabolism if appropriate. Reversibility tests. If necessary, observation of local irritation at injection sites. For injectable biochemical drug: pyrogen test, foreign protein test, allergy test.
Overdose intoxication:	If clinical trial is proposed for a special kind of drug with high toxicity and narrow margin of safety, antidote for overdose intoxication desirable.

Reproduction studies

General remarks

Dose levels:	2 or 3 plus control group. Highest dose should produce slight toxic reactions, low dose should be 2 to 3 times therapeutic dose.
Route:	Normally same as proposed for use in man, oral administration via stomach tube.

Reproduction studies

Species:	One or more.
Sex:	M and F.
Age:	Sexually mature animals.
Number of animals:	If mice or rats are used: at least 20 of each sex per group.
Administration period:	M 60, F 14 days prior to mating. Once day 0 of pregnancy has been ascertained, pregnant F to be treated throughout organogenesis.
Experimental procedure:	Treated M and F to be placed in same cage for up to 2 weeks. If necessary: treated M and untreated F or vice versa may be mated. During mating F examined for presence of vaginal plug and sperm for determination of positive mating. Preg-

China

	nant F to be autopsied one day before expected delivery. Autopsy of all treated M and F where copulation unsuccessful. Histopathology if appropriate.
Variables:	Detection of pregnancy, resorptions, stillbirths, development of live fetuses in uterus, morphological examination including internal organs and bones. If appropriate: histological and histochemical examination.

Teratogenicity

Species:	At least one (usually mouse or rat).
Number of animals:	15 to 20 pregnant mice or rats, 8-12 pregnant rabbits per group.
Route:	Normally same as proposed for use in man. Oral administration via stomach tube.
Dose levels:	At least 2 or 3 plus control group. Highest dose may induce slight toxic reactions, lowest dose should be a multiple of proposed therapeutic dose.
Administration period:	Throughout fetal organogenesis.
Experimental procedure:	All treated animals should be sacrificed at final stage of gestation.
Variables:	Detection of pregnancy, resorptions, stillbirths, development of live fetuses in uterus, morphological examination including internal organs and bones. Histological and histochemical examination if appropriate.
Exception:	a) For some new drugs observation of F1 until adulthood. In such cases 10 additional pregnant F required per group. b) F should be allowed to litter normally. F1: observation of neonatal survival, growth and development, behavior, reproductive function, abnormal signs. If appropriate long-term observation of F1: reproductive function, gestation, parturition and general health of F2.

Perinatal studies

Species:	Mouse, rat or rabbit.
Number of animals:	15-20 pregnant mice or rats, 8 to 12 pregnant rabbits per group.
Administration period:	Late stage of pregnancy throughout lactation.
Experimental procedure:	F should be allowed to litter normally. If appropriate long-term observation of F1: reproductive function, gestation, parturition and general health of F2.

China

Carcinogenicity

General remarks

In selecting species and strains, resistance of animals to infectious diseases, life-span, incidence of spontaneous tumor and susceptibility to carcinogens should be considered. Animals used for preliminary and carcinogenicity tests of a particular drug should be of same species and strain from same animal house. Administration of drug to rodents should begin as soon as possible after weaning.

1) Preliminary carcinogenicity test

Species:	Rodents.
Sex:	M and F.
Number of animals:	10 of each sex per group.
Route:	Same as in carcinogenicity test.
Dose levels:	3 plus control. Highest dose in carcinogenicity tests should be based on result of subacute toxicity test. Compared with control group, this dose should induce less than 10 % depression of body weight gain, cause no death and no significant change in general condition.
Administration period:	Continuously for 90 days. For drugs with chronic accumulation effect longer administration period required.
Experimental procedure:	When drug is given mixed with food or drinking water, consumption of food or drinking water should be measured regularly for calculation of amount of drug taken.
Variables:	Daily observation of general condition, weekly measurement of body weight. Necropsy and pathological examination of dead animals and those surviving conclusion of test. Histopathology of organs showing lesions or abnormalities.

2) Carcinogenicity test

Sex:	M and F.
Number of animals:	50 of each sex per test group and control group.
Dose levels:	At least 3.
Control groups:	Solvent or vehicle control group, blank control group desirable.
Administration period:	Rats at least 24 months, mice or hamsters at least 18 months.
Variables:	Daily observation of general signs. Weekly measurement of body weight and food intake during first 13 weeks, once every 4 weeks thereafter. Necropsy at conclusion of test. If blood disorder diagnosed, count of peripheral white and red blood cells. Whenever tumor, or lesion suspected to be a tumor, is found by gross observation, histopathology of all organs. If no tumors are found, histopathology of all organs in 1/3 to 1/2 of animals in high-dose group.

China

Observation indicators:	Survival rate should be more than 50 % at the end of 24 months for rats, 18 months for mice and hamsters.
Evaluation:	Result considered positive if

– tumor is present in test group, absent in control group,
– tumor is present in test and control groups, but incidence of tumor is higher in test group than in control group;
– tumor incidence is essentially identical in test and control group, however, tumor formation is more rapid in test group than in control group.

Presence of clear carcinogenic effect in one species implies drug may, potentially, be carcinogenic in man. Negative results from all animals (preferably 2 species) imply that drug is non-carcinogenic.

Mutagenicity

3 kinds of tests, according to chemical structure, physico-chemical properties and genetic end-point effects of drug:

1) Reverse mutation assay

Microbe strains:	4 (TA97, TA98, TA100, TA102) of histidine defective Salmonella typhimurium or some WP2 strains of E. coli.
Dose levels:	Highest dose depends on bacterial toxicity and solubility; usually up to 5 mg/plate. At least 5 dose levels, if fewer, explanation should be given.
Metabolic activation:	In vitro assay in presence of mammalian liver microsomal enzymes (S9) pre-treated with inducer. Parallel assay on the system without S9.
Control groups:	Solvent as negative, known mutagen as positive control.
Evaluation:	Results positive, when increase in number of reverse mutation colonies is dose-dependent or when such an increase at one particular dose level is reproducible.

2) Chromosomal aberration assay in mammalian cell culture

Cells:	Primary culture mammalian cells or continuous cell lines.
Dose levels:	At least 3, highest dose should produce 50 % inhibition of cell growth, if not dosage level should be justified.
Exposure times:	Usually chromosome preparation after cells have been exposed to drug for 24 and 48 hours.
Metabolic activation:	Appropriate method should be used.
Control groups:	Solvent as negative, known mutagen as positive control.
Microscopic examination:	100 metaphase cells at each concentration should be examined for chromosome structural aberration and appearance of multiploids.
Evaluation:	Results positive, when appearance frequency of chromosomal aberrations is higher in treated groups than in negative

controls, and when response is dose-related. Frequency of appearance and type of abnormal cells should be indicated.

3) In vivo test

Normally, only micronucleus test necessary, but for drugs acting on the reproductive system dominant lethal test should be carried out.

a) Micronucleus test in rodents

Species:	Usually mouse.
Age:	Sexually mature.
Sex:	M and F.
Number of animals:	5 of each sex per group or at least 6 M per group.
Dose levels:	At least 3, highest dose 1/2 LD50, if not, dose level should be justified.
Route:	P.o. and/or i.p.
Administration:	Single dose. Administration may be repeated if necessary.
Control groups:	Solvent as negative control and known mutagen as positive control.
Specimen preparation:	18 to 30 or 12 to 72 hours after drug administration animals should be sacrificed, bone marrow removed for centrifugation and smears stained with Giemsa stain or acridine orange.
Microscopic examination:	1000 polychromatic erythrocytes from each animal should be examined to determine incidence of cells with micronuclei and the ratio of polychromatic to normochromatic erythrocytes.

Evaluation: Results positive when increased incidence of cells with micronuclei compared with control group is significant and dose-dependent, or when such an increase at one particular dose level is reproducible.

b) Dominant lethal test in rodents

Species:	Usually mouse.
Age:	Sexually mature.
Number of animals:	15 M per group.
Dose levels:	3, however, 1 or 2 may be used in preliminary tests. Highest dose should be based on maximum tolerated dose ensuring 100% survival of animals after continuous administration of drug for 30 days.
Route:	P.o. or i.p.
Administrtation period:	Daily for 5 days or 6 weeks, or one single dose.
Mating:	Treated M with non-treated F successively at appropriate intervals. Mating time to depend on administration method:

	animals given single dose or one daily dose for 5 days, mating time up to 6 weeks after final administration; animals dosed continuously for 6 weeks, mating time up to one week after final administration.
Control groups:	Solvent as negative control and substance known to induce positive dominant lethal effect as positive control. Positive control may be omitted if such a test has already been performed in same laboratory, using same line of animal species.
Variables:	Laparotomy of F during final stage of pregnancy, determination of number of embryonic implantations in uterus, live and dead fetuses, and non-implantations. For determination of dominant lethal rate, average survival of fetuses in pregnant mice of test and negative control group.
Evaluation:	Dominant lethal effects positive, when increase in number of dead fetuses and non-implantations, or decrease in total number of live fetuses and embryonic implantations is significant, and dose-related. Dominant lethal rate (DL) is defined as follows:

$$DL(\%) = \left(1 - \frac{\text{average survival rate of fetuses in test group}}{\text{average survival rate of fetuses in negative control group}}\right) \times 100$$

Local toxicity tests

Requirement:	Drugs used for local application.
Method:	These drugs are usually absorbable, therefore, preliminary local absorption test should be performed, followed by systemic toxicity tests appropriate to the extent of local absorption. Local irritation tests should be performed at site of application, development of and recovery from irritation (i.e. inflammation) should be monitored by gross and microscopic examination of tissues.

a) Dermatological drugs

Species:	Rats or guinea pigs, usually adult animals. Adolescent animals for tests of drugs topically used on baby skin.
Dose levels:	At least 3.
Number of animals:	Not less than 3 in each group to allow observation of any toxic reactions restricted to one particular dose level.
Observation period:	Usually not more than 14 days after final application.
Method:	Dermal toxicity and skin sensitization tests should be performed on intact and damaged skin.

b) Nasal drops and inhalants

Species:	Rats or guinea pigs.

Concentration groups:	At least 3.
Sex:	M and F.
Number of animals:	10 in each group (5 M and 5 F).
Exposure time:	Not less than 4 hours.
Observation period:	Usually 14 days.
Method:	Toxicity test and test for local irritation in respiratory tracts (including lungs) should be performed.

c) Eye drops

Species:	Preferably rabbits.
Number of animals:	At least 3.
Drug application:	0.1 ml per application for drug in solution form. Not more than 100 mg per application for ointments.
Observation period:	Usually up to 21 days after final administration, for evaluation of reversibility of toxic reactions.
Variables:	Observation of local irritation of conjunctiva and eyeball.

d) Preparations used topically on rectum and vagina

Method:	Local irritation test and local toxicity test should be performed at site of application.

Drug dependence tests
Direct method

Species:	At least one species of small animals (rats or mice) and one species of large animals (monkeys).
Application period:	Drug administered to animals at least twice a day.
Dosage levels:	Gradually increased – without allowing appearance of toxic reactions – to maximum tolerated dose.
Withdrawal of drug:	After continuous administration for at least 3 months.
Variables:	Animals observed for appearance of abstinence syndrome: convulsions and other evident excitement symptoms.
Method:	For drugs with possible opiate effects, competitive antagonist may be used to precipitate abstinence syndrome. In this case, period of continuous administration should not be too long (3-7 days), but number of administrations per day should be increased. Normally the maximum tolerated dose should be reached within a short period, then an antagonist injected to observe whether abstinence syndrome is precipitated.

China

Substitution test

Method: Drug with knwon dependence-producing action is administered to animals daily. Once onset of physical dependence has been established by presence of abstinence syndrome, test drug is administered to determine whether it relieves abstinence syndrome.

Costa Rica

Document reviewed:

COSTA RICA: Ministerio de Salud, Consejo Tecnico de Inscripciones, Departamento Drogas Estupefacientes, Controles y Registros. Reglamento de Inscripciones y Propaganda de Medicamentos y Cosméticos. Costa Rica. Not dated.

Address of Regulatory Agency:

Ministerio de Salud, Departamento de Drogas, Estupefacientes, Controles y Registros, Apartado 10123, San José, Costa Rica.

The relevant paragraphs are reproduced below in English translation:

«Requirements for registration of new drugs:

Article 42. New drugs are considered those which have never been used or evaluated as therapeutic agents in this country, as well as those which are already known, but will be used in new and different pharmacological applications and therapeutic indications.

Article 43 The following information must be provided:
– distribution of drug in organism
– absorption and effects of drug on different organs and systems
– drug metabolism and possible pharmacological action of metabolites
– endocrinological and teratological actions
– effects on fertility, sucklings and lactation
– permeability of placenta by drug
– excretion
– microbiological tests if necessary
– pharmacological tests in animals
– bioavailability if possible
– precautions and contraindications
– acute, subacute and chronic toxicity studies
– comparison of pharmacological action in humans and animals, value of such a comparison and tests used to determine it
– tests to determine therapeutical safety
– systemic and local safety
– determination of dose range for humans
– pediatric studies if necessary
– if product to be used over long periods of time, additional studies of long-term effects

Costa Rica

Article 44 When drug or one of its components is produced abroad, all clinical experiments supporting the application for registration must be performed in the countries where the drug is then registered. In addition, results must be published in recognized scientific journals.

Article 45 The data shall include comparative studies with drugs of similar therapeutic action.»

Republic of Cyprus

Note:

THE REPUBLIC OF CYPRUS has not yet published any laws or regulations governing safety testing of new drugs and diagnostics prior to clinical investigation and marketing, nor any administrative rules for obtaining a licence to conduct clinical trials. However, all new drugs must be registered in accordance with the provisions of the Drugs (Control of Quality, Supply and Prices) Law 6/67. (Letter fom the Pharmaceutical Services of the Ministry of Health of the Republic of Cypurs, Nicosia, November 28, 1987.)

Address of Regulatory Agency:

The Drugs Council, Ministry of Health, Nicosia – Cyprus.

Denmark

Note:

DENMARK uses the **Nordic Guidlines** for clinical testing, drug applications, evaluation reports on proprietary medicinal products and registration of allergen preparations.

DENMARK uses the **EEC II Guidelines** of November 1983 for repeated dose toxicity studies, reproduction studies, carcinogenicity studies, pharmacokinetic and metabolic studies in the safety evaluation of new drugs in animals.

DENMARK uses the **EEC IV Guidelines** of March 1987 for single dose toxicity studies and mutagenicity studies.

Address of Regulatory Agency:

Sundhedsstyrelsens farmaceutiske laboratorium, Frederikssundsvey 378, DK-2700 Bronshoj, Denmark.

Egypt

Documents reviewed:

EGYPT I: Documents Required for the Registration of Pharmaceutical Specialities.(Not dated.)

EGYPT II: Ministry of Health: Decision Number 56 for the year 1985 for arrangements concerning performing the clinical studies and the import of some drugs that are not registered in the country. February 3, 1985.

Address of Regulatory Agency:

Director of the General Administration for Drug Registration, the Central Administration for Pharmaceutical Affairs, Ministry of Health, Cairo, Egypt.

Note:

There are no government guidelines concerning preclinical safety tests. However, the scientific file should include the results of such tests. These data are subjected to evaluation by a scientific committee.

EGYPT I: Documents Required for the Registration of Pharmaceutical Specialities. (Note dated.)

The relevant paragraphs are reproduced below in English translation:
«3. Certificate of origin and free sale issued from the Ministry of Health in the country of origin, legalized by the Egyptian Embassy or Consulate in that country, including : a) Name and address of the manufacturer
        b) Name and strength of the product, name and quantity of active ingredients
        c) Evidence that product is freely available in its country of origin under same name and with same composition.
10. A full scientific file for the new product including formula, data from pharmacological, toxicological and clinical studies, etc... and stability data.»
The other paragraphs pertain to the form of application, analytical data and pricing information.

EGYPT II: Ministry of Health: Decision Number 56 for the Year 1985 for arrangements concerning performing the clinical studies and the import of some drugs that are not registered in the country. February 3, 1985.

The relevant paragraph is reproduced below in English translation:
«d) The pharmaceutical preparation should already be registerd and marketed in the country of origin or in other countries that are known to have drug control laboratories (e.g. U.S.A., Sweden, Switzerland).»

Federal Republic of Germany (FRG)

FRG uses the **EEC-Guidelines** and the «**Arzneimittelprüfrichtlinien**».

Document reviewed:

FRG: Arzneimittelprüfrichtlinien nach Paragraph 26 Arzneimittelgesetz. Draft December 12, 1986 (Published in: Pharm. Ind. **49**, No. 1, 1987).

Address of Regulatory Agency:

Institut für Arzneimittel, Bundesgesundheitsamt, Postfach 33 00 13, D-1000 Berlin 33.

Summary of Toxicological Guidelines:

Acute toxicity

Species:	2 rodents, unless a single species of rodents can be justified. Only in special cases should mammalian species other than rodents be used.
Determination of LD50:	Precise determination usually not required.
Route:	At least 2, one as proposed for use in man, unless one single route can be justified.
Variables:	Functional and morphological defects of organs, organ systems and application sites. Time of onset and duration of effects, reversibility/irreversibility and interactions of tested drug and other drugs.

Subchronic and chronic toxicity

Species:	Usually 2 mammals, one a non-rodent, unless one single species can be justified.
Duration:	Several days to 6 months; in special cases several years.
Dose levels:	To be justified.
Route:	As proposed for use in man.
Size of groups:	No exact numbers are given. Should be sufficient to allow determination of all toxicologically relevant effects and dose-effect relationship.
Variables:	Growth and development of animal, behavior, hematology, urinalysis, clinical chemistry, organ function, autopsy, histopathology. Time of onset, duration and reversibility of toxic effects. Evaluation of risk of toxic effects in man.

FRG

Reproduction study

Scope of study:	Effects on or interference with – development of the conceptus – copulatory behavior – fertilization – development of embryo and fetus – parturition – postnatal development.
Species:	One rodent; for treatment during organogenesis one additional non-rodent. Primates only in special cases (to be justified). Choice of species to depend on clinical data for man (pharmacokinetics).
Dose levels:	3. – Highest dose: to produce toxic signs in M or F parent (e.g. body weight loss), but no effect on nursing behavior of dam. – Lowest dose: either to produce a pharmacodynamic effect in animal, or to attain a blood concentration necessary to produce a pharmacodynamic effect in man, or a dose corresponding to that proposed for use in man.
Route:	As proposed for use in man.
Administration:	– From spermatogenesis up to implantation of embryo – Throughout period of organogenesis – Throughout fetal development up to end of lactation
Variables:	– Number of: pregnant F, corpora lutea, implantation sites, resorptions, live and dead fetuses, abnormalities. – Duration of pregnancy and parturition. – Postnatal development and mortality of pups. – If necessary: effects on development and behavior of progeny.

Carcinogenic potential

Requirements:	When – chemical structure, results of earlier tests or other data, give rise to suspicion of carcinogenic effects – substances are likely to be administered continuously or periodically over a prolonged period of life, or – substances proved to have a long retention time.
Species:	One rodent. Under special circumstances (e.g. differences in pharmacokinetics and metabolism between animal and man) an additional species (choice to be justified).
Duration of administration: Route:	To be determined in the light of proposed use in man and known reactions of species and strain (choice to be justified).
Dose levels:	3. – Highest dose: to produce minimal toxic effects, but pre-

FRG

	ferably to produce sub-toxic effects only.
	– Lowest dose: similar to dose proposed for use in man and if possible to produce pharmacological effect in animal.
Variables:	If tumors are observed, frequency, type of tumor and time of onset.

Mutagenic potential

Scope of study:	To detect gene and chromosome mutations.
Species:	To be selected according to specific characteristics of substance to be tested.
Method:	In vitro procedures and usually one in vivo test. Tests to be selected according to specific characteristics of substance.

Local toxicity

Requirements:	Drugs intended for application to skin and mucous membranes.
Method:	Drug should be applied on large area of intact and broken skin and mucous membrane.
Information on:	Penetration, permeation, systemic effects. Local effect after repeated applications. Sensitizing properties of drug and its components.

Finland

Note:

FINLAND uses the **Nordic Guidelines**.

Address of Regulatory Agency:

Lääkintöhallitus/Medicinalstyrelsen, Apteekkitoimisto/Apoteksbyran, Siltasaarenkatu 18 A, PL 224, SF-00531 Helsinki 53, Finland.

France

Document reviewed:

FRANCE: Ministère de la Santé. Protocole applicable aux essais toxicologiques et pharmacologiques des spécialités pharmaceutiques. 10 août, 1976, modifié par arrêté du 2 octobre, 1985. – FRANCE also accepts current **EEC-Guidelines**.

Address:

Ministère des Affaires Sociales et de l'Emploi, Direction de la Pharmacie et du Médicament, Mission des Affaires Internationales et Communautaires, 1, Place de Fontenoy, F-75700 Paris.

Summary of Toxicological Guidelines:

Acute toxicity, or single dose effects

Species:	At least 2 mammalian species of a specified strain.
Sex:	Equal numbers of M and F.
Route:	At least 2, one identical or similar to route proposed for use in man, one to assure absorption of product.
Observation period:	Not less than one week, to be determined by the investigator.
Determination of LD:	LD50 with 95 % confidence limits, if possible.
Combinations:	Tests to demonstrate potentiation or new toxic effects in presence of several active components.
Variables:	Observed signs, including local tolerance.

Subacute and chronic toxicity, or repeated dose toxicity

Species:	2 mammalian species, one a non-rodent.	
Duration:	Single dose treatment in man:	2 to 4 weeks.
	Short-term use in man:	2 to 4 weeks.
	Long-term use in man:	3 to 6 months.
Route:	To be chosen by investigator, but future therapeutic use and possibility of absorption should be taken into consideration.	
Administration frequency:	Must be clearly indicated.	
Dose levels:	High dose need not be selected to produce toxic effects, since margin of safety can be determined using lower doses.To be chosen by investigator, justification should be supplied.	
Variables:	Behavior, growth, hematology, organ functions (especially organs of excretion), autopsy, histopathology.	
Combinations:	Tests may be simplified for new combinations of known	

Experimental detail:	components if no potentiation or new toxic effects are found in acute and subacute tests. To be chosen by investigator, justification to be supplied. An excipient used for the first time in therapy should be treated like an active component.

Teratogenesis or fetal toxicity

Requirement:	Omission of tests must be justified (e.g. if drugs are not proposed to be given to women of childbearing age).
Species:	At least 2, possibly 3; rabbit of a strain responsive to known teratogens, and rat or mouse of specified strains recommended.
Methods:	According to current state of teratological science and such as to attain statistical significance. (Number of animals, dose levels, stage of pregnancy of administration, criteria for evaluation of results not specified.)

Reproduction studies

Requirement:	If data from other tests suggest a potential for anti-fertility effects or adverse effects on offspring.
Methods:	According to prevailing state of science. Not specified.

Carcinogenesis

Requirement:	Close chemical analogy to substance known to have carcinogenic or co-carcinogenic activity. Substances with suspicious results after long-term tests. Substances with suspicious results after mutagenicity or other carcinogenicity tests. Substances proposed to be used over a long period of life.
Methods:	According to prevailing state of science. Not specified.

Mutagenicity

Requirement:	For every new substance to reveal mutagenic effects on genetic material causing permanent and inheritable changes on offspring.
Methods:	According to current state of science. Not specified.

Local toxicity

Requirement:	Where a pharmaceutical speciality is intended for topical use.
Scope of study:	Investigation of absorption of product, also for possible use on broken skin.
Method:	If absorption under these conditions is negligible, repeated dose toxicity tests, fetal toxicity tests and studies of reproductive function may be omitted.

France

If resorption is demonstrated during clinical experimentation, toxicity tests shall be carried out on animals, and where necessary, fetal toxicity tests.

In all cases tests of local tolerance after repeated application shall be carried out and include histological examinations. Possibility of sensitization shall be investigated and any carcinogenic potential.

German Democratic Republik (GDR)

Document reviewed:

GDR: Gesetzblatt der Deutschen Demokratischen Republik, Teil I Nr. 37, Berlin, December 10, 1986.

Address of Regulatory Agency:

Institut für Arzneimittelwesen der DDR, Grosse Seestrasse 4, Berlin, 1120.

The relevant paragraph is reproduced below in English translation:

«3. Pharmacological-toxicological study: This study shall characterize the effects of the substance including tolerability. This is to be achieved by tests on animals and other biological systems. Where possible, tests on animals should be replaced by suitable alternative tests. The characterization of the effects of antigen- and antibody-containing preparations and of preparations of lymphocytes shall be based on immunological-toxicological tests. Products equivalent to drugs which are to be used by humans shall be tested as to their tolerability and functional quality.»

Greece

Note:

GREECE uses the **EEC Guidelines**. The form of the application must correspond to the: Commission of the European Communities. Notice to Applicants for Marketing Authorizations for Proprietary Medicinal Products in the Member States of the European Community on the Use of the New Multi-State Procedure Created by Council Directive 83/570/EEC, April 1986. This document explains the contents and structure of a submission to EEC countries.

Address of Regulatory Agency:

E.O.F. National Drug Organization, 4, Voulis St., Athens 10 562, Greece.

Hong Kong

Document reviewed:

HONG KONG: Pharmacy and Poisons Ordinance, Cap. 138: Registration of Pharmaceutical Products/Substances. Notes for the Guidance of Applicants. June 1985.

Address of Regulatory Agency:

Pharmacy and Poisons Board, Medical and Health Department, 1/F., Centre Point Building, 181-185, Gloucester Road, Wanchai, Hong Kong.

Note:

There are no specific rules or guidelines for safety testing of new drugs and diagnostics prior to clinical investigation and marketing in Hong Kong, and the above document is only a general guide and should not be treated as a complete or authoritative statement of the law on any particular case. However, for information, the relevant paragraphs concerning registration are summarized below in English translation:

«The following information is required for evaluation by the Pharmacy and Poisons Board before a licence to authorize a clinical trial or medicinal test can be granted:

a) A sample of the drug or diagnostic and a copy of the protocol for the clinical trial together with a written request from a local clinical investigator concerning the clinical trial.
b) Documents or research papers demonstrating the safety of the new drug or diagnostic for clinical study.
c) Documents, if any, showing the clinical studies or registration status of the new drug or diagnostic in the country of origin and/or any other countries.

Clinical papers from the country of origin and from at least one or two advanced countries demonstrating the safety, efficacy and quality of the new dosage forms of approved drugs must be submitted for evaluation.

Registration is required by law in Hong Kong for the marketing of a drug or diagnostic which is a pharmaceutical product or medicine. The criteria for registration are safety, efficacy and quality. For a new drug or diagnostic, detailed clinical studies from both the country of origin and some advanced countries are required for evaluation. The registering authority may require further information from an applicant for drug/diagnostic registration if it thinks fit.»

Hungary

Document reviewed:

HUNGARY: The National Institute of Pharmacy. Guidelines for Safety Testing of New Drugs. Summary of draft, Budapest, 1987.

Address of Regulatory Agency:

National Institute of Pharmacy, Zrinyi u. 3., H-1051 Budapest, Hungary.

Note:

The detailed guidelines, which have been in force since January 1, 1988, do not yet exist in an English version.

Summary of Toxicological Guidelines:

Acute toxicity

Species:	2 rodents, and one non-rodent.
Route:	Different routes of administration.
LD50:	Determination of exact LD50 in non-rodents not required.

Long-term, subacute and chronic toxicity

Duration:	Normally 6 months; depending on intended clinical use.

Reproduction and teratology

Requirements: Segment I – fertility tests – only required, if in long-term toxicological and special endocrinological studies signs of toxic effect on spermatogenesis, oogenesis or on ovulation process have been observed. Teratological data from segment I are needed when women of childbearing age will take part in the phase I and II clinical studies.
Segment II investigations only required for drugs which will be used during perinatal period or lactation.

Carcinogenicity

Requirements: When
– drug proved to be mutagenic
– compound or its metabolites show some structural similarity to known carcinogenic agents
– drug caused bone marrow toxicity, spermatotoxicity, or increased tumor incidence in long-term toxicological studies
– drug showed some teratogenic effects

Hungary

– the National Institute of Pharmacy orders the performance of these investigations

Mutagenicity

Methods: At least 1 in vivo and 2 in vitro tests (no specific tests are recommended).

Requirements: When drug
– is intended for use in chronic treatment
– shows some structural similarity to known mutagenic agents
– gave indications of possible mutagenic effects in long-term toxicity studies.

Other studies

No details of special studies for tissue irritation, skin sensitization, local toleration etc. are included in the above summary, but will be given in the new guidelines.

Iceland

Note:

ICELAND uses the **Nordic Guidelines**.

Address of Regulatory Agency:

Heilbrigdis- og Tryggingamalaraduneytid, Lyfjanefnd, Laugavegur 116, IS-105 Reykjavik, Iceland.

India

Document reviewed:
INDIA: Central Drug Standard Control Organization. Guidelines on Introduction of New Drugs. New Delhi, 1985.

Address of Regulatory Agency:
The Drugs Controller, Directorate General of Health Services, Ministry of Health & Family Welfare, Nirman Bhawan, New Delhi – 110 001, India.

Summary of Toxicological Guidelines:

General remarks
Animal toxicity data available from other countries are acceptable and do not need to be repeated/duplicated in India.

Acute toxicity

Species:	At least 2, usually mice and rats.
Route:	Same as intended for humans; in addition at least one other to ensuring systemic absorption of drug.
Observation period:	Up to 72 hrs after parenteral and up to 7 days after oral administration.
Observations:	Symptoms, signs, mode of death, results of macroscopic and microscopic examinations when necessary.
Determination of LD50:	LD50 should be determined with 95 % confidence limits; if LD50 cannot be determined, explanation should be given.

Long-term toxicity

Species:	At least 2 mammals, one a non-rodent. Where metabolism of the drug in a particular species is known to resemble that in humans, this species should be included.
Duration:	Depending on whether the application is for marketing permission or for clinical trials, and in the latter case, on phase of trials (see Appendix).
Route:	As intended for clinical use.
Administration schedule:	7 days per week.
Dose levels:	Highest dose should produce observable toxicity. Intermediate dose should cause some signs, but not gross toxicity or death, and may be logarithmic mean of highest and lowest dose. Lowest dose should not cause observable toxicity, but should be comparable to intended therapeutic dose or a multiple of it, e.g. 2.5x.

India

Control groups:	A vehicle control group must be included.							
Variables:	Behavioral, physiological, biochemical, and microscopic observations.							
Number of animals:	Minimum numbers on which data should be available:							

Number of animals:

Group	2-6 weeks				7-26 weeks			
	Rodents (rats)		Non-rodents (dogs)		Rodents (rats)		Non-rodents (dogs)	
	M	F	M	F	M	F	M	F
Control	6-10	6-10	2-3	2-3	15-30	15-30	4-6	4-6
Low dose	6-10	6-10	2-3	2-3	15-30	15-30	4-6	4-6
Intermediate dose	6-10	6-10	2-3	2-3	15-20	15-20	4-6	4-6
High dose	6-10	6-10	2-3	2-3	15-30	15-30	4-6	4-6

Reproduction studies

Requirements:	For drugs proposed to be used in women of child-bearing age.
Species:	2, one a non-rodent, if possible.

a) Fertility studies

Sex:	M and F.
Administration period:	Beginning a sufficient period before mating. In F treatment should be continued after mating, and pregnant F should be treated throughout pregnancy.
Dose levels:	Highest dose should not affect general health or growth of animals.
Route:	Same as for therapeutic use.
Number of animals:	Control and treated groups should be of similar size, containing at least 20 pregnant F and at least 8 pregnant F in control groups of rodents and non-rodents respectively.
Variables:	Thorough examination of the litters from both groups, included spontaneous abortions.

b) Teratogenicity studies

Administration period:	Throughout period of organogenesis.
Dose levels:	3. One should cause minimal maternal toxicity, one should be same as proposed for clinical use.
Route:	Same as proposed for clinical use.
Number of animals:	Rodents: 20 pregnant F, non-rodents: 12 pregnant F per dose group.
Variables:	Number of implantation sites, resorptions, number of fetuses with their sexes, weights, and malformations.

c) Perinatal studies

Administration period:	Throughout last third of pregnancy, and through lactation to weaning. Dose which causes low fetal loss should be continued throughout lactation to weaning.
Number of animals:	Control and each treated group at least 12 pregnant F.
Experimental procedure:	Weanlings should be sacrificed.
Variables:	Macroscopic examinations, autopsy and histopathology where necessary.

Local toxicity

Requirements:	When drug is proposed to be used topically in humans.
Species:	Guinea-pigs or rabbits.
Experimental procedure:	Drug should be applied to appropriate site in suitable species. If drug is absorbed, appropriate systemic toxicity studies required. (For details see Appendix).

Carcinogenicity and mutagenicity

Requirements:	If drug or its metabolites are related to known carcinogen. When nature and action of drug is such as to suggest a mutagenic/carcinogenic potential.

Carcinogenicity

Species:	At least 2. Species should not have a high incidence of spontaneous tumors and should preferably metabolize drug in same manner as humans.
Dose levels:	At least 3. Highest dose should be sublethal but cause observable toxicity. Intermediate dose may be logarithmic mean of highest and lowest doses. Lowest dose should be similar to intended therapeutic dose or a multiple of it, e.g. 2.5x.
Administration schedule:	7 days per week.
Control group:	Must be included.
Variables:	Macroscopic changes observed at autopsy and detailed histopathology.

India

Appendix

Route of Administration	Duration of Human Administration	Phase	Long-term Toxicity Requirements
Oral or parenteral or transdermal (systemic)	single dose or several doses in 1 day	I-III MP	2 sp; 2 wk
	up to 2 wk	I; II	2 sp; up to 4 wk
		III; MP	2 sp; up to 3 mo
	up to 3 mo	I; II	2 sp; up to 4 wk
		III	2 sp; 3 mo
		MP	2 sp; up to 6 mo
	over 3 mo	I; II	2 sp; 3 mo
		III; MP	2 sp; 6 mo
Inhalation (general anesthetics)		I – III MP	4 sp; 5 d (3h/d)
Aerosols	repeated or chronic use	I; II	1-2 sp; 3 exp
		III	1-2 sp; up to 6 wk (2 exp/d)
		MP	1-2sp; 24wk (2exp/d)
Dermal	short-term or long-term application	I; II	1 sp; single 24 h exp, then 2 wk observation
		III; MP	1 sp; number and duraion of applications commensurate with duration of use
Ocular or otic or nasal	single or multiple applications	I; II	Irritation test; graded doses
		III	1 sp; 3 wk; daily application as in clinical use
		MP	1 sp; number and duration of applications commensurate with duration of use
Vaginal or rectal	single or multiple applications	I; II III; MP	1 sp; number and duration of applications commensurate with duration of use

Abbreviations: sp = species; wk = week; d = day; h = hour, mo = month; exp = exposure; MP = Marketing Permission; I, II, III = phases of clinical trial

Italy

Document reviewed:
ITALY: Gazetta Ufficiale della Republica Italiana. No. 238, September 9, 1977.

Address of Regulatory Agency:
Ministero della Sanità, il Direttore Generale del Servizio Farmaceutico, Viale della Civiltà Romana 7, I-00144 Roma, Italia.

Summary of Toxicological Guidelines:

Acute toxicity

Species:	At least 2 mammalian species, one a non-rodent.
Sex:	M and F.
Route:	At least 2, one identical with or similar to that proposed for human use, the other to guarantee absorption of substance.
Observation period:	To depend on duration of action of the new drug.
Determination of LD:	LD50 with confidence limit in at least one animal species.
Variables:	Description of toxic signs.

Subacute or repeated dose toxicity

Species:	2, one a non-rodent.
Duration:	At least 12 weeks. 3 to 4 weeks for those drugs which, in pilot clinical trials, will be given not more than twice.
Route:	As proposed for therapeutic use.
Dose levels:	At least 3, except in exceptional and justified cases. Highest dose to cause toxic effects and kill at least some of the treated animals.
Variables:	Behavior, weight change, hematology, function of excretory organs, autopsy, histopathology.

Chronic or long-term toxicity

Duration:	At least 6 months.
Method:	Same as in subacute toxicity study.

Fetal toxicity

Species:	Rabbit (strain known to be sensitive to teratogens) and another animal of specified strain.

Reproduction studies
Fertility

Species:	One or more.

Italy

Administration:	Start: a sufficient time before pairing M and F to cover gametogenesis. F: throughout gestation.
Route:	As proposed for use in man.
Dose levels:	In accordance with use in man.
Experimental procedure:	One part of F hysterectomized shortly before parturition, other part of F spontaneous delivery.
Variables:	Observation of pups of treated dams, weight curve, neurological and behavioral development. Test of reproductive ability: allow one M and one F per litter to mate (with a partner from another litter).

Peri-postnatal toxicity

Treatment:	During period after embryogenesis and during lactation period.
Variables:	Same as in fertility study.

Carcinogenicity

Requirement:	– If results of chronic toxicity tests show suspicious biochemical and/or histological changes. – If substance shows close structural analogy to substances known to have carcinogenic activity.

Two levels of tests:

First level tests:
1. Direct oncogenic effect on especially sensitive substrates.

Types of tests:	a) Topical effect: s.c. administration to mouse or rat. In case of insoluble products application may be single. For soluble and rapidly absorbed products application shall be repeated on five consecutive days. Observation period until natural death of the animals. b) General oncogenic effect: chronic treatment, oral and/or i.p. according to the nature of the substance in mouse or rat strains with high response to carcinogens.
Dose levels:	Maximum dose levels compatible with a long-term experiment should be applied.
Observation period:	To the spontaneous death of the animals or in a positive case, until result is significant.

2. Perinatal oncogenic effect.

Species:	2, at least one a rodent.
Sex:	F.
Administration period:	Daily throughout embryogenesis and lactation.
Dose levels:	As proposed for use in man.
Route:	As proposed for use in man.
Observation period:	Pups should be observed for 24 months, then sacrificed for macro- and microscopic examination of various organs.

Italy

Second level tests:

Requirement:	When first level tests cause suspicion and when the characteristics of the drug justify it.
Species:	At least 2, one a rodent strain with low response to carcinogens.
Sex:	Equal numbers of M and F.
Duration:	At least 18 months of treatment from weaning.
Route:	P.o., in diet or drinking water or according to the nature of the substance. In special cases a second route based on clinical use.
Dose levels:	2, one the maximum tolerated dose, one a fraction thereof, e.g. 1/2 or 1/4.
Number of animals:	Large enough to permit reasonable statistical treatment.
Control group:	At least same number of animals as in treatment groups.
Observation period:	To the natural death of the animal.
Evaluation:	According to WHO Technical Report No. 426.

Mutagenicity

Test procedures:	In vitro tests with bacteria, eukaryotic microorganisms both with and without metabolic activation systems. Repair tests, e.g. unscheduled DNA synthesis.

Japan

Document reviewed:

JAPAN I: Toxicity Test Guideline 1984. Collection of Notifications Related to the Pharmaceutical Affairs Law (IV).
JAPAN II: Guideline for quality assurance on drug products obtained by cell culture (draft). March 31, 1987.

Address of Regulatory Agency:

Pharmaceutical Affairs Bureau, Ministry of Health and Welfare, 2-2, Kasumigaseki 1-chome, Chiyoda-ku, Tokyo 100, Japan.

Summary of Toxicological Guidelines:
General remarks

Experimental animals: When acute, subacute, and chronic toxicity studies are performed on a substance, it is desirable that animals of the same species and strain be used. Generally, mice and rats are used as rodents, and dogs and monkeys as non-rodents.

Extent of testing: To depend on duration of clinical application:

TABLE:
Administration Frequency or Period

Period of Clinical Application	Acute Toxicity	Subacute Toxicity	Chronic Toxicity
Drugs to be administered once	once	28 days	not required
Drugs to be administered for a period exceeding one week and not exceeding 4 weeks	once	90 days	not required
Drugs to be administered exceeding one week and up to four weeks	once	28 days	6 months
Drugs to be administered for more than four weeks	once	90 days	1 year

Acute toxicity with rodents

Species: At least 2, using healthy adult animals, normally mice and rats.
Sex: M and F.
Number of animals: At least 5 of each sex per group.
Administration: Single as a rule.

Japan

Route:	In principle oral and parenteral, including expected clinical route. If the latter is not applicable to animals, other appropriate routes. Oral administration should be made forcibly as a rule, in which case animals should be fasted for a certain time before administration. In case of parenteral administration, at least 2 routes desirable.
Dose levels / LD50:	Sufficient numbers for determination of LD50 values for each sex. Generally, at least 5 groups are employed, and the LD50 is calculated by probit analysis, etc. If toxicity of the substance is too low to determine LD, a technically applicable maximum dose should be employed as highest dose.
Observation period:	2 weeks in principle.
Experimental procedure:	Daily observation of general signs, measurement of body weights 3 times during observation period. At termination of observation period (or at time of death) autopsies and gross observations of all organs and tissues of all animals. Organ weights and histopathological examination of any organ showing gross changes.
Note:	In 1987, **new draft guidelines** for acute toxicity tests were issued as follows:
Species:	At least 2 (1 non-rodent. but not rabbit) desirable.
Sex:	M and F at least in 1 species.
Number of animals:	At least 5 per group in rodents, 2 per group in non-rodents.
Route:	Rodents: oral and parenteral, including the expected clinical route.
	If drug is used intravenously only, test only by intravenous route.
	Non-rodents: expected clinical route only.
Dose levels:	Rodents: sufficient number to determine approximate lethal dose (LD5O), (at least 3).
	Non-rodents: sufficient number for observation of clear toxic signs (at least 2).
Upper limit dose:	Oral: 2000 mg/kg.
Observation period:	2 weeks usually.
Observations:	Type, grade, time of appearance, progression, and reversibility of toxic signs.
	Autopsy of all animals, and histopathology of any organ showing gross changes.

Acute toxicity with non-rodents

Species:	At least one (usually dogs or monkeys).

Japan

Number of animals:	At least 2 per group.
Route:	In accordance with expected clinical route. Oral administration may be made forcibly, or by ad lib. intake mixed with food or dissolved in drinking water.
Dose levels:	At least 2, sufficient for determination of approximate LD.
Administration:	Single as a rule.
Observation period:	2 weeks as a rule.
Experimental procedure:	Daily observation of general signs, measurement of body weights 3 times during observation period, clinical laboratory tests if necessary. Autopsies and gross examination of all organs and tissues at termination of observation period or at time of death. Histopathological examinations and measurement of organ weights if necessary.

Subacute toxicity in rodents

Species:	At least one, using healthy adult animals. Same as in acute toxicity.
Sex:	M and F.
Number of animals:	At least 10 of each sex per group. When study includes a specific test imposing a heavy burden on the animals, interim sacrifice or recovery testing, the animals for such use should be asigned beforehand.
Administration period:	28-90 days (see Table on page 101), 7 days a week.
Route:	In accordance with expected clinical route, as a rule. Oral administration may be made forcibly, or by ad lib. intake mixed with food or dissolved in drinking water, in which case actual intake of substance should be calculated from food or water intake.
Dose levels:	At least 3 plus control group for each sex. Sufficient dosages and number of dose groups to determine toxic and no-effect dose levels on the basis of results of acute toxicity study or of a preliminary short term study with consecutive administration. A toxic dose should cause death in some of the animals or apparent toxic signs, and a non-effect dose should cause no toxic signs in any of the animals.
Control groups:	Negative control group plus negative control groups for additives and vehicles alone. Non-treated control group desirable.
Experimental procedure:	Daily observation of all animals for general signs, measurement of food intake and body weights once a week. At least once during administration period, urinalysis, ophthalmological examination and other clinical laboratory tests. Autopsies and gross examinations of all organs and tissues,

Japan

body weight and histopathological examination on all animals which died, or were moribund. Hematological examinations and blood chemical analysis of the latter animals. Identical examinations should be performed on surviving animals at the conclusion of the administration period.

Experimental details for
subacute and chronic toxicity tests for rodents and non-rodents:

Test items:	Urinalysis: urinary volume, specific gravity, pH, occult blood, total protein, glucose, ketone bodies, urobilinogen, bilirubin and sediment.
	Ophthalmology: cornea, conjunctiva, sclera, iris and fundus.
Histopathology:	Normally on following organs and tissues: skin, mammary gland, lymph nodes, submaxillary gland, sternum, femur (with bone marrow), thymus, trachea, lung and bronchi, heart, thyroid gland and parathyroid gland, tongue, esophagus, stomach and duodenum, small intenstine, large intestine, liver, pancreas, spleen, kidney, adrenal gland, urinary bladder, epididymis, prostate, testis, ovary, uterus, vagina, brain, pituitary gland, spinal cord, eye, Harder's gland, and other organs and tissues showing gross alterations.
Blood tests:	Hematological examinations and blood chemical analyses should include as many test items as possible. Methods and units of measurement should be those commonly used internationally.

Chronic toxicity in rodents

Species:	At least one of healthy adult animals.
Sex:	M and F the same weeks of age.
Number of animals:	At least 20 of each sex per group.
Administration period:	6-12 months (see Table on page 101), 7 days a week as a rule.
Route:	In accordance with expected clinical route as a rule. Oral administration can be made forcibly, or by ad lib. intake mixed with food or dissolved in drinking water.
Dose levels:	At least 3 plus control group for each sex. Same as in subacute toxicity study.
Control groups:	Negative control group plus negative control groups for additives and vehicles alone. Non-treated control group desirable.
Experimental procedure:	Same as in subacute toxicity.

Subacute toxicity with non-rodents

Species:	At least one (normally dogs or monkeys).
Sex:	M and F.

Japan

Number of animals:	At least 3 of each sex per group.
Route:	In accordance with expected clinical route, as a rule. Same as in acute toxicity study.
Dose levels:	At least 3 plus control group for each sex. Same as in subacute toxicity study with rodents.
Control groups:	Negative control group plus negative control groups for vehicles, additives and capsules alone.
Administration period:	28 or 90 days (see Table first page 101), 7 days a week.
Experimental procedure:	Daily observation of general signs, measurement of food intake and body weights once a week. During administration period, urinalysis, ophthalmological examination and other clinical laboratory tests. Autopsies and gross examinations of organs and tissues, body weight and histopathological examination of all animals which died, or were moribund. Hematological examinations and blood chemical analyses of the latter animals. Identical examinations should be performed on surviving animals at the conclusion of the administration period.

Chronic toxicity in non-rodents

Species:	At least one (normally dogs or monkeys).
Sex:	M and F.
Number of animals:	At least 4 of each sex per group.
Route:	As proposed for use in man.
Dose levels:	At least 3 plus control for each sex.
Control groups:	Negative control group plus negative control group for vehicles, additives and capsules alone.
Administration period:	6 months or 1 year (see Table page 101), 7 days a week.
Experimental procedure:	Same as in subacute toxicity study.

Reproduction study

Requirement:	All drugs to be administered prior to and during pregnancy and at the perinatal and lactation periods. More detailed studies may be required on drugs with suspected effects on fertility or if given to many pregnant women.

General remarks:

Experimental animals:	Species and strains should be selected in the light of reproductive information such as fertility, rate of spontaneous malformations and sensitivity to substances known to affect reproduction. Selection of species and strains with low rates of spontaneous malformations desirable. Animals used in

Japan

Route:	studies a), b) and c) should be of same strain and species. – Preferably, mammals having relatively well understood general metabolic machanisms (which should be similar to those of humans) and which may be readily employed in this type of study, should be used. – When species other than rats, mice or rabbits are employed, sufficient number of animals for evaluation of the results should be used. For studies a) and c): Oral administration can be made forcibly, or by ad lib. intake mixed with food or dissolved in drinking water. Forced administration is superior to other methods because fixed dose levels are applied without fail. If expected clinical route is not applicable, another appropiate method may be employed.
Dose levels:	Highest dose should cause some toxic signs such as decreased food intake or inhibition of body weight gain. When no toxic signs appear with maximum applicable dose, such dose should serve as highest dose. Intermediate dose(s) should be geometric mean(s) of highest and lowest dose. Lowest dose should not cause any adverse effect in parent animals, fetuses or young. Dose levels should include a dose that exhibits pharmacological effects in animals used or is not far different from the expected usual dose in clinical practice.

a) Administration tests prior to and in the early stages of pregnancy

Species:	Both sexes of at least one (rat or mouse).
Age:	M: at least 40 days, F: sexually mature.
Number of animals:	At least 20 of each sex per group should be used for mating.
Route:	In accordance with expected clinical route as a rule.
Dose levels:	At least 3 plus control.
Control groups:	Negative control group and, if necessary, positive or comparative control group. Referral should be made to background data obtained previously to supplement the results in the negative control group. Negative control groups for vehicles and additives alone. Positive control group receiving a substance known to have potent reproductive toxicity. Comparative control group receiving an available drug with similar chemical structure or pharmacological effects.
Administration period:	For rats and mice: M: from 60 or more days daily until successful mating. F: for at least 14 days before mating daily until beginning of fetal organogenesis (mouse day 6, rat day 7). Examples of administration periods in F after successful copulation (day 0 = day when copulation confirmed): In rats,

Japan

	days 0-7, in mice days 0-6. Copulation and fertility index should be calculated for F and M.
Experimental procedure:	During administration period observation for mortality and general signs; measurement of food intake and body weights.
Mating:	Treated M with treated F, daily observation for successful copulation. Mating period between same M and F 2 weeks. If necessary, mating of treated F with non-treated M, daily observation for successful copulation.
Variables:	When copulation is successful autopsy of all F at term: number of corpora lutea, successful pregnancy, dead fetuses, etc. Gross examination of organs and tissues of dams. Autopsies of M and F where copulation unsuccessful.

b) Administration tests during period of fetal organogenesis

Species:	F of at least one rodent (mouse or rat) and one non-rodent (rabbit).
Number of animals:	Animals with successful pregnancy: each group at least 30 rats or mice and at least 12 rabbits.
Route:	In accordance with expected clinical route as a rule.
Dose levels:	At least 3 plus control.
Control groups:	Negative control and positive or comparative control group if necessary. Negative control group for vehicles and additives alone. Positive control receiving a substance known to have potent reproductive toxicity and comparative control receiving an available drug with similar chemical or pharmacological effects.
Administration period:	Continuously throughout organogenic period (mouse day 6 to 15, rat day 7 to 17, rabbit day 6 to 18). Examples of administration periods in F after successful copulation: In rats, days 7-17, in mice, days 6-15, in rabbits, days 6-18. Copulation and fertility index should be calculated for F and M.
Experimental procedure:	Dams of 2/3 of rodents and of all rabbits autopsied in final stages of pregnancy. Dams of 1/3 of rodents should be allowed to deliver and nurse their young. Gestation index should be calculated. Examination of dams for abnormality on delivery.
Variables:	During administration period examination of all dams for mortality and general signs. Measurement of body weights and food intake. Body weight measurement and morphological examination of live fetuses. Findings for estimating time of death in utero should be noted. On live fetuses in late stages of pregnancy examination of external and internal organs and tissues, morphology in the skeleton and ossification with cleared and stained skeletal specimens.

Japan

Number, mortality, sex, and external alterations of newborns, measurement of body weights. Also growth and development (behavior), any abnormal symptoms, reproductive functions, etc. Autopsy and gross observations of organs and tissues of treated dams at appropriate time. Examination of second litters if necessary.

c) Administration tests during perinatal and lactation periods.

Species:	F of at least one (mouse or rat) as selected for b).
Number of animals:	Dams of rats and mice with successful pregnancy: at least 20 per group.
Route:	In accordance with expected clinical route as a rule.
Dose levels:	At least 3 plus control group.
Control groups:	As in b).
Administration period:	Continuously from approximately the end of organogenic period until weaning (mouse day 15 to day 21 pp, rat day 17 to day 21 pp, rabbit day 18 to day 21 pp). Examples of administration periods in F after successful copulation: In rats, day 17 to 21 after delivery; in mice, day 15 to 21 after delivery. Copulation and fertility index should be calculated for F and M.
Experimental procedure:	Examination of dams for mortality and general signs, measurement of food intake and body weights. All F: spontaneous delivery and nursing of their young. Variables: As in b).

Carcinogenicity

Requirement: If carcinogenicity is suspected from chemical structure or pharmacological effects, or results of chronic or other toxicity studies. If clinical use of substance is expected to be prolonged.

General remarks:

Experimental animals: Species and strains should be selected in the light of resistance to infectious disease, life span, spontaneous tumor rate, sensitivity to known carcinogens, etc. – Animals of same species and strains should be used for preliminary and full-scale carcinogenicity studies of a particular substance.

I Preliminary carcinogenicity study

Requirement: To determine the dose levels for carcinogenicity studies, if no reliable data are available.

Acute toxicity

Study is performed with a small number of animals to determine highest dose in subacute toxicity study.

Japan

Subacute toxicity

Study is performed to determine highest dose in carcinogenicity study.

Species:	At least 2 (at present usually rats, mice, or hamsters) of the same age, not older than 6 weeks. Study should be started as soon as possible after weaning.
Sex:	M and F.
Number of animals:	10 of each sex per group.
Route:	Same as in the carcinogenicity study. Oral administration may be made forcibly, or by ad lib. intake mixed with food or dissolved in drinking water. – When substance is administered mixed with food, concentration of substance in food should not exceed 5 %
Dose levels:	At least 3 plus control groups for each sex. It is desirable, that the common ratio of dose levels be 2 or 3. Highest dose should cause some toxic effect. When no toxic signs appear with maximum applicable dose, such a dose should serve as highest dose. Intermediate dose should be geometric mean of highest and lowest dose level. Lowest dose should not cause any toxic effect. When substance is given mixed with food or dissolved or in drinking water, food and water intake should be measured in order to calculate actual intake of substance. Purity and stability of any impurities in substance should be analyzed qualitatively and quantitatively as far as practicable before and at appropriate time during study.
Administration period:	90 days, 7 days a week. If substance has delayed toxic effects or cumulative effects, longer period may be necessary.
Experimental procedure:	Daily observation for general signs, measurement of body weights once a week. Autopsies and gross examinations of organs and tissues of dead animals, and of surviving animals at the conclusion of administration period. Histopathology of organs and tissues showing gross changes.
Results:	Highest dose in carcinogenicity study should inhibit body weight gain by less than 10%, and should cause neither death due to toxic effects nor remarkable changes in the general signs of the animals in the subacute toxicity study. A specific highest dose should be selected for each species and sex.

II Carcinogenicity study

Species:	At least 2 (at present usually rats, mice, or hamsters) of same age, not older than 6 weeks. Study should commence as soon as possible after weaning.
Sex:	M and F.
Number of animals:	At least 50 of each sex per group. Allocation to each group at random.

Japan

Route:	In accordance with expected clinical route. Oral administration may be made forcibly, or by ad lib. intake mixed with food or dissolved in drinking water. – When substance is given mixed with food, concentration of substance should not exceed 5 %.
Dose levels:	At least 3 plus control for each sex. Highest dose should be determined from result of subacute toxicity study. Intermediate dose should be geometric mean of highest and lowest dose. Lowest dose should cause some pharmacological effect or should be in accordance with expected clinical dose. Lowest dose should be more than 10 % of highest dose. However, when lowest dose is very different from expected clinical dose, another dose of less than 10 % of highest dose may be employed. When substance is administered mixed with food or in water, food or water intake should be measured in order to determine actual intake of substance. Purity and stability of any impurities in the substance should be analyzed qualitatively and quantitatively as far as practicable before and at appropriate times during study.
Control groups:	Negative control plus negative control group for vehicles or additives alone.
Administration period:	At least 24 months for rats (max. 30 months) and at least 18 months for mice and hamsters (max. 24 months). Administration 7 days a week. When forced administration is employed, administration may be performed 5 or 6 days a week.
Experimental period:	Termination either at or 1 to 3 months after end of administration period, 30 months for rats and 24 months for mice and hamsters at the longest. Termination of study when cumulative mortality reaches 75 % in lowest dose group or in control. Then surviving animals should be sacrificed and study terminated. Mortality due to causes other than tumors should be within 50 % after 24 months of administration for rats and 18 months for mice and hamsters. Loss of animals due to autolysis, cannibalism and problems in husbandry should not exceed 10 % in any group. Isolation or sacrifice for autopsy should be considered for animals found prostrate or moribund during study. Daily observation of general signs, measurement of body weights of all animals. Autopsies, gross examinations and histopathology of all organs and tissues of animals which died or were moribund. Identical examinations should be performed on surviving animals at the conclusion of the administration period. Histopathology of: Skin, mammary gland, lymph node, sali-

vary gland, sternum, vertebrae or femur, thymus, trachea, lung and bronchi, heart, thyroid gland and parathyroid gland, tongue, esophagus, stomach and duodenum, small intestine, large intestine, liver, pancreas, spleen, kidney, adrenal gland, urinary bladder, epididymis, prostate, testis, ovary, uterus, vagina, eye ball, brain, pituitary gland, spinal cord, and other organs or tissues with tumor lesions found during gross examinations.

Detection of changes diagnostic of imminent tumor-formation should be included in description of lesions. At sacrifice, count of peripheral RBC and WBC in blood collected at that time, preparation of smears.

Examination of smears in preparations suggestive of blood disorder such as anemia, increase of lymph nodes, swelling of liver and spleen etc.

Mutagenicity

Requirement: All new drugs should be subjected to mutagenicity studies with gene mutation and chromosomal aberration as indices. Bacterial reversion test (I), in vitro chromosomal aberration test (II), in vivo micronucleus test (III). When mutagenicity is suspected from I or II, performance of III desirable.

Further tests should be performed where their necessity is implied by the results of the above test methods, or other tests of safety or efficacy. A list of tests applicable at present is given in the original guidelines.

Test methods: **I Bacterial reversion test**:

Strains: Several strains of Salmonella typhimurium and Escherichia coli.

Dose levels: 5 or 6 plus control groups. Substance should be tested at maximum dose of 5 mg per plate as a rule. If substance shows antibacterial activity, highest dose should be the dose where anitbacterial effect is observed.

Control groups: Negative and positive control group. A solvent group as negative control. Authentic mutagens for positive control groups both in presence and absence of S9 mix.

Metabolic activation: Simultaneous performance of tests both in presence and absence of S9 mix. S9 should be prepared from liver of a mammal previously treated with appropriate inducer of drug metabolic enzymes.

Test methods: Preincubation method or plate incorporation method. When substance has antibacterial activity, such as antibacterial drugs, mutation frequency should be calculated from number of surviving bacteria and revertants, determined after incubation of substance with bacterial test strains, washing of cells and resuspension.

Japan

Presentation of results:	Real number and mean value of revertants in tables.

II In vitro chromosomal aberration test:

Cells:	One of primary or established cell lines of mammalian (including human) cells in culture. Cells with high sensitivity should be used where possible.
Dose levels:	At least 3 plus control groups. Highest concentration should be determined to produce 50 % inhibition of cell growth. When no cytotoxic effect is observed, concentration should not exceed 10mM or maximum solubility.
Control groups:	Negative and positive control groups. A solvent group as negative control. A substance known to cause chromosomal aberrations as positive control.
Metabolic activation:	It is desirable to employ an appropriate metabolic activation method concurrently. S9 mix should be prepared from liver of a mammal previously treated with appropriate inducer of drug metabolic enzymes.
Experimental procedure:	Chromosome preparation at appropriate time after treatment. Examination for structural chromosomal aberrations and polyploid cells on 100 metaphase cells per group. In describing morphological abnormalities, types of structural abnormality in chromosomes or chromatids should be made clear.
Presentation of results:	Incidence of cells with chromosomal aberration or frequency of chromosomal aberrations per cell in tables.

III In vivo micronucleus test:

Note:	The chromosomal aberration test in bone marrow cells of rodents may be used instead.
Species:	One rodent (e.g. mouse).
Sex:	M should be used as a rule, but F may be used where drug is clinically used in F only.
Number of animals:	At least 5 per group.
Route:	I.p. or as expected clinical route. Oral administration should be made forcibly in principle.
Dose levels:	At least 3 plus control groups. Maximum tolerated dose should be determined by single (or consecutive) administration in a preliminary test, if necessary. Highest dose should cause some toxic signs such as inhibition of body weight gain, if possible. If maximum applicable dose does not cause any toxic signs, that dose should be employed as highest dose.
Control groups:	Negative and positive control groups. Negative control groups for vehicles and additives alone. Positive control group receiving a substance known to induce micronuclei.

Japan

Administration:	Single as a rule. If necessary consecutive administration. In latter case administration should be made 4 or 5 times.
Experimental procedure:	Sacrifice of all animals at appropriate time after administration, preparation of smears of bone marrow. Normally, animals should be sacrificed at a specific time (18-30 hrs) after administration of substance for preparation of specimens. Chronological preparation (several times in 24-72 hrs) may be employed. A preliminary test should be performed if necessary. Period of highest sensitivity should be selected from results. Observation of incidence of micronuclei in 1,000 polychromatic erythrocytes per animal. Calculation of ratios of polychromatic and normochromatic erythrocytes. Incidence of reticulocytes may be substituted for incidence of polychromatic erythrocytes.
Presentation of results:	Incidence of polychromatic erythrocytes with micronuclei and ratio of polychromatic and normochromatic erythrocytes should be presented in tables and charts.

Biotechnology Products

Document reviewed:

JAPAN II: Guideline for quality assurance on drug products obtained by cell culture (draft). March 31, 1987.

This draft document defines the various drug products obtained by cell culture methods and indicates the information required on methods of manufacture and control of biotechnology products. See also pages 186–187.

Toxicity testing

General remarks:

The document points out that it is at this time not possible nor reasonable to establish uniform standards and methods of studies. Therefore, the guideline provides general principles for the performance of scientifically pertinent studies and stresses the necessity of a «case by case approach».

Species:	As far as possible, animal species showing physiological or pharmacological responses to the active components should be selected. Reasons for species selection should be stated.
Routes:	As similar as possible to those intended for clinical use.
Frequency and duration:	As similar as possible to those intended for clinical use.
Special procedure:	When repeated administrations are made, antibody production in test animals should be monitored. Studies should, whenever possible, continue even when antibodies are produced.

Japan

Exceptions: Part of toxicity tests may be omitted if active ingredients of drug product obtained by cell culture are identical to those of product derived from humans, and if results of toxicity studies of such materials are available.

Acute toxicity
These studies to be conducted in all cases.
Species: At least 2.

Subacute toxicity
Requirement: Not required for vaccines used only once or a few times.

Chronic toxicity
Requirement: Studies should be conducted when necessary, but may be omitted on reasonable grounds.

Reproduction
Requirement: Studies should be conducted when necessary, but may be omitted on reasonable grounds.

Special requirement: If compound contains active components having structures different from those of components derived from humans or is likely to be administered to pregnant women or women of reproductive age, these studies are obligatory. Pharmaceuticals suspected of causing abortions should be tested in primates.

Mutagenicity
Requirement: Studies should be conducted as a rule.
Test procedures: Studies must be performed when necessary, but may be omitted on reasonable grounds.

Dependence and local irritation
Requirement: Studies must be performed when necessary, but may be omitted for reasonable causes.

Antigenicity tests
Requirement: Necessary for products administered for long periods of time and those having chemical structure apparently different from those of components derived from humans.

Impurities
Requirement: Impurities derived from cell media: verification methods. Substances related to active components should be tested for specific antibody production. Possible interaction with active component should be considered.
These tests may be omitted on reasonable grounds.

Japan

Pyrogen test
Requirement: Pyrogen tests using rabbits or other test methods should be conducted.

Special activities
Requirement: Special studies may be necessary for compounds with particular physiological activity, e.g. those affecting the immune system.
Monoclonal antibodies should be studied for their ability to cross react with antigens similar to but different from the target antigens.

Kuwait

Document reviewed:

KUWAIT: Letter from the Ministry of Public Health. October 24, 1987.

Address of Regulatory Agency:

Ministry of Public Health, Drug Control and Registration Centre, P.O. Box 5, Safat, Kuwait – Arabian Gulf.

The relevant sections concerning safety testing are reproduced below (citation from ministerial decree No. 302/80):
«Before clinical evaluation of a drug, product safety testing is carried out in the pharmacology department, and the LD50 of the active drug substance is taken into consideration.
The factors that can effect the safety testing carried on laboratory animals are: the strain, sex, age, the caging of the animals, the consumed food and water, the room temperature. These factors are carefully controlled. The choice of animal species is an important consideration. Usually the testing is carried out in at least four species, one being non-rodent and depends on the dosage form under investigation. In addition to the safety testing, there are a variety of other tests which are routinely performed depending on the drug substance and the dosage form, such as hemolysis testing, irritation tests (eye, skin, muscle, venous, vaginal and rectal irritation, skin-sensitization) and tetsts on oral dosage forms.» etc.

Note:

Preclinical safety tests are the responsibility of sponsor company prior to conducting clinical trials.

Hemolysis testing
Requirement: All parenteral drugs.
Species: Dog.
Procedure: I.v. injection over a 30 sec. period. Determination of plasma hemoglobin 1 minute later.

Irritation tests
Eye irritation test
Requirement: Ophthalmic preparations and any other topical or cosmetic formulation.
Species: Rabbit.
Number of animals: 3.
Dosage: 0.1 ml, or 0.1 g.

Kuwait

Procedure: Instillation in conjunctival sac. Observation 1, 2, 4, 24, 48 and 72 h later.

Skin irritation

Species: Rabbit
Number of animals: 3.
Dosage: 0.1 ml, or 0.1 g.
Procedure: Application on normal and abraded skin. Observation 24 and 72 h later.

Muscle irritation

Species: Rabbit or rat.
Number of animals: 9 per dose level.
Dosage: 1.0 ml and 0.1 ml.
Procedure: I.m. injection. Sacrifice 3 animals after 24, 48 and 72 h. Gross examination of injection sites.

Venous irritation

Species: Dog or rabbit (ear vein).
Procedure: Observation of vein after slow i.v. injection.

Vaginal and rectal irritation

Species: Rabbit or rat.
Procedure: Place suppositories in vagina and rectum. Sacrifice animals 24 h later. Examine for erythmea and edema.

Skin sensitization

Species: Guinea pig.
Procedure: Place compound on shaved back of 10-20 guinea pigs every other day for 3 weeks. Grade application site for erythema and edema.

Luxembourg

Note:

Currently, there are no government guidelines concerning preclinical and clinical safety tests.

LUXEMBOURG uses the **EEC guidelines**.

Address of Regulatory Agency:

Grand-Duche de Luxembourg, Direction de la Santé, Division de la Pharmacie et des Médicaments, 10, rue C.M. Spoo, 2546 Luxenbourg.

Malaysia

Document reviewed:

MALAYSIA: Drug Control Authority Ministry of Health, Malaysia. Control of Drugs and Cosmetics Regulations 1984.

Address of Regulatory Agency:

Drug Control Authority, National Pharmaceutical Control Laboratory, Ministry of Health, Jalan University, P.O. Box 319, Petaling Jaya, Selangor, Malaysia.

Summary of Toxicological Guidelines:

General remarks:	In at least one species drug should have an activity related to expected therapeutic effect.
	Species to be selected on basis of metabolic similarity to man.
	Drug to be given in the vehicle intended for therapeutic application or final pharmaceutical formulation.
	New vehicle or excipient should be investigated in same manner as active ingredients.
	Possibility of toxic reactions following systemic absorption should be explored for drugs intended for topical application.
	For substances in combination, potentiation or novel toxic effects to be determined.
	Positive as well as negative results must be reported.
	If product intended for use in children, weanlings also to be studied. Similarly for geriatric products.
	Comparative studies using other standard drugs and extrapolation of results to man where possible.

Acute toxicity

Species:	3, one a non-rodent.
Sex:	M and F.
Route:	3 or more, including that proposed for use in man and one to ensure systemic absorption, i.e. i.v., i.m., or s.c.
Dose levels:	Several, logarithmically spaced. Highest dose should be toxic and kill some animals.
Obervation period:	Period during which signs are present or may be expected; at least one week after administration.
LD50:	Must be determined.
Variables:	Food consumption, body weight, toxic signs, changes in appearance and behavior, locomotion, tissue reactions, ophthalmic, respiratory and cardiovascular effects.

Malaysia

Autopsy: All animals dying during experiment.

Subacute / chronic toxicity

Purpose: To study:
– potential toxicity of drug/ingredient during prolonged administration,
– therapeutic margin in animal species tested,
– whether toxic effects are reversible or irreversible,
– which organs, tissues, or systems are affected and the effects.

Species: 2, one a non-rodent.
Sex: M and F.
Duration: Determined by proposed duration in man and pharmacokinetics of drug.
Observation period: Period during which signs are present or may be expected; at least one week after administration.
Variables: See acute toxicity. Additional parameter: hematology, biochemistry and urinalysis.
Autopsy: All animals. Determination of cause of death where possible. Histopathology.

Reproduction studies / Teratogenicity

Species: 2 mammalian, one a non-rodent.
Number of animals: Sufficient to enable statistical analysis.
Dose levels: 3. Highest dose may be toxic but not lethal to mother. Lowest dose should be below toxic dose and close to effective dose in animal or to the proposed therapeutic dose.
Route: As proposed for use in man. Other routes if necessary.
Timing and duration: Appropriate to the toxic effect studied.
Control groups: Adequate control groups in all studies. Ideally, one group to be left alone after conception and another group to be handled in the same way as the experimental group, without receiving the drug.

Teratogenicity / Embryotoxicity

General principles: see WHO publication «Principles for the Testing of Drugs for Teratogenicity», Technical Report Series No. 364 (1967). Reports must contain information on species used, route, dosing schedule/duration.
Variables: Examination of fetuses: number dead or alive, weight, sex, external and internal malformations, most sensitive stage. Examination of placenta: weight, histological examination, examination of uterus. Examiation of postnatal animals: Some offspring should be allowed to survive until sexual

Malaysia

maturity to determine whether developmental derangements have affected biochemical or functional, including behavioral parameters.

Fertility and general reproduction studies

Purpose: To elucidate influence on fertility and general reproductive ability of M and F and the female reproductive cycle. Effects on gonadal function, estrus cycle, mating behavior, fecundation, early stages of gestation and whole reproductive process including teratogenesis, late stages of gestation, parturition, lactation and weaning, growth, development, fertility and behavior of F_1 generation.

Species:
Sex:
Route: to be mentioned.
Dosing schedule/duration:
Experimental procedure:

In fertility studies:
Some F should be sacrificed at appropriate stage of gestation. Record of following information: Number of corpora lutea, implantation sites and resorptions, number, weight and sex of indivuidual fetuses, skeletal and/or visceral abnormalities in fetuses.

Remainder of treated animals should be allowed to litter normally and the young observed up to weaning and sexual maturity. Number of young, malformation, weight at birth, survival rate of young, effect on duration of pregnancy, stillbirths, litter size, etc. should be noted. The young should be observed for: a) late effects of drug on progeny (auditory, visual and behavioral functions), b) reproductive function in progeny by allowing at least one M and one F from each litter of treated animals to breed.

Perinatal and postnatal studies

Administration period: Period of gestation during which substance was not administered in fertility and general reproduction studies (see above) and during last third of pregnancy, throughout period of lactation up to weaning.

Species:
Route: to be mentioned
Dosing schedule/duration:
Experimental procedure: Treated dams should be allowed to litter spontaneously. Record following information: effects on mother, parturition, fetus or neonate, lactation and growth of weanling, and late effects on offspring.

Malaysia

Carcinogenicity

Requirement: Where substance or its metabolite has a chemical structure or pharmacological properties that suggest carcinogenic potential/resemble known carcinogens.

Where substance causes concern as a result of: a) some specific aspects of its biological action, b) its pattern of toxicity or retention.

Where substance would be used in man continuously for long periods or have frequent intermittent usage, as in treatment of chronic illness.

General principles: See WHO publication «Principles for the Testing and Evaluation of Drugs for Carcinogenicity», Technical Report Series No. 426 (1969). Reports must contain information on species used, route, sex, dose levels, duration, variables.

Mutagenicity

Requirement: All drugs should be evaluated. Priority for testing compounds that are chemically, biochemically or pharmacologically related to known or suspected mutagens.

Compounds that exhibit certain toxic effects in animals, such as: a) depression of bone marrow at tolerated doses, b) inhibition of spermatogenesis or oogenesis at maximum tolerated doses, c) inhibition of mitosis at maximum tolerated doses, d) teratogenic effects at maximum tolerated doses, e) carcinogenic effects, f) causation of sterility or semi-sterility in reproduction studies, g) stimulation or inhibition of growth or synthetic activity of a specific organ, cell or virus, h) inhibition of immune response at maximum tolerated dose.

Drugs that are often used over a period of years particularly in children and young adults.

Drugs that are prescribed to a large proportion of the population.

Drugs used for general prophylaxis.

Drugs subject to widespread abuse.

Drugs that come in contact with sperms in high concentrations, e.g. substances used for sperm preservation and vaginal contraceptives.

Biol. substances that contain live microorganisms or affect DNA.

General principles: See WHO publication «Evaluation and Testing of Drugs for Mutagenicity: Principle and Problems», Technical Report Series No. 482 (1971). Reports must contain information on species or media used; sex, where applicable; route, where applicable; dosing schedule/ duration; variables observed.

Malaysia

Dependence liability studies

Requirements: Drugs structurally related to compounds known to have dependence liability in man. Drugs acting on CNS e.g. analgesics, depressants, hallucinogens, stimulants.

General principles: See WHO publication «Evaluation of Dependence-Producing Drugs», Technical Report Series No. 287 (1964). Reports must contain summary of results of in-vitro/animal studies for tolerance, physical and psychic dependence effects, mentioning species or media used; sex, where applicable; route; dosing schedule/duration.

Drug combinations (where applicable)

Requirements: Where product contains 2 or more active ingredients, data on pharmacological and toxicological profile of combination as well as individual components.

Information on: Modification of: activity of individual components, toxicity of individual components.

The Netherlands

Note:

THE NETHERLANDS use the **EEC Guidelines**.

Address of Regulatory Agency:

Committee for the Evaluation of Medicines, P.O. Box 5811, 22 HV Rijswijk, Holland.

New Zealand

Document reviewed:

NEW ZEALAND: Department of Health New Zealand. Medicine Distribution, a Guide for Importers, Manufactureres, Distributors and Suppliers of Medicines, Medical Devices and Related Products in New Zealand. The Medicines Act 1981, Medicines & Benefits, 1987.

Address of Regulatory Agency:

Department of Health, Head Office, Macarthy Trust Building, Lambton Quay, Wellington, New Zealand.

Summary of Toxicological Guidelines:

General

Medicine used should be identical to that proposed for clinical use and generally final preparation should also be used.

Acute toxicity

Species:	At least 2 mammals, one a non-rodent.
Route:	As proposed for clinical use, plus p.o. and by injection in at least one species.
Determination of LD:	Quantitative evaluation of LD should be provided in a suitable species, but high level of precision is not required.
Dose levels:	Description of effects of highest tolerated dose.
Number of animals:	Sufficient number of animals to enable valid conclusions to be drawn.
Variables:	Toxic effects and their time of appearance, changes in behavior and appearance of animals, histopathological changes.

Prolonged toxicity

Species:	At least 2 mammalian, one a non-rodent.
Sex:	M and F.
Dose levels:	Several appropriate dose levels should be used.
Duration of tests:	Longer than duration of proposed clinical use.
Number of animals:	Sufficient number of animals to enable valid conclusions to be drawn.
Variables:	Any observed toxic signs and histopathological changes.

Reproduction and fertility

Scope of study:	Data should be provided about any adverse effects on fertility, general reproductive ability of M and F, and F reproductive cycle.

New Zealand

Species:	At least one mammal.
Dose levels:	Several appropriate dose levels should be used.
Number of animals:	Sufficient number of animals to enable valid conclusions to be drawn.

Teratogenicity

Scope of study:	Data should be provided about any embryotoxic and teratogenic effects.
Species:	At least 2 mammals.
Dose levels:	Several appropriate dose levels should be used.
Number of animals:	Sufficient number of animals to enable valid conclusions to be drawn.

Peri- and post-natal toxicity

Scope of study:	Data should be provided about any adverse peri- and post-natal effects.
Species:	At least one mammal.
Dose levels:	Several appropriate dose levels should be used.
Number of animals:	Sufficient number of animals to enable valid conclusions to be drawn.

Carcinogenicity and mutagenicity

Requirements:	When medicine and/or its metabolite(s) are related to any known carcinogenic and/or mutagenic substance. When drug is to be administered over a prolonged period or to children.
Dose levels:	Several appropriate dose levels should be used.
Number of animals:	Sufficient number of animals to enable valid conclusions to be drawn.
Experimental procedure:	In vitro and in vivo mutagenicity tests may be necessary to provide complementary evidence.
Publications:	Recent publications on carcinogenicity and mutagenicity should be provided.

Norway

Note:

NORWAY uses the **Nordic Guidelines.**

Address of Regulatory Agency:

Statens Legemiddelkontroll, Sven Oftedals vei 6, N-0950 Oslo, Norway.

Republic of the Philippines

Note:

THE REPUBLIC OF THE PHILIPPINES is presently in the process of formulating guidelines for the registration of new drugs and diagnostics. (Letter of the Bureau of Food and Drugs, Dept. of Health, Metro Manila, December 15, 1987).

Address of Regulatory Agency:

Bureau of Food and Drugs, Alabang, Muntinlupa, Metro Manila, Republic of the Philippines.

Poland

Document reviewed:

POLAND: Directives of the Minister of Health and Social Welfare of 3rd December 1979 as regards carrying out laboratory testing and clinical trials of finished drug dosage forms and sanitary materials (published in: Off. Gazette of the Ministry of Health and Social Welfare No. 14).

Address of Regulatory Agency:

Department of Pharmacy, Ministry of Health and Social Welfare, 38/40 Dluga Street, 00-238 Warszawa, Poland.

Summary of Toxicological Guidelines:

General remarks

The Drug Commission is authorized to expand the pharmacological investigation with investigation of metabolism and also to present a more detailed specification for the mode of testing.

Acute toxicity

Species:	2 mammals.
Route:	P.o. and parenteral.
Cumulative toxicity:	Determination of cumulative toxicity in 1 species using 1 administration route.

Subacute toxicity

Species:	2, same as used in acute toxicity.
Route:	P.o. and parenteral.
Duration:	At least 3 weeks.
Dose levels:	Quantitative and qualitative determination of pharmacological properties and calculation of maximum tolerated dose.

Chronic toxicity

Species:	2.
Route:	1, as proposed for use in man.
Duration:	At least 2 months. Drug Commission is authorized to specify duration.

Pharmacokinetic tests

Species:	2.
Route:	2.
Variables:	Determination of bioavailability and pharmacokinetics.

Poland

Safety pharmacology
Determination of pharmacological properties that could give information on potential side-effects in man.

Teratogenicity
Requirement: When chemical structure indicates that compound may become a teratogen.
Species: 3.

Carcinogenicity / mutagenicity and other effects
In justifiable cases Drug Commission is authorized to expand pharmacological investigation to include investigation of carcinogenic and mutagenic activity, metabolism, fertility, development of tolerance and drug dependence, sensitizing properties, etc.

Portugal

Note:

The PORTUGESE guidelines could not be sent, as they are presently under revision (letter from the Ministry of Health, January 14, 1988).

Address of Regulatory Agency:

Direção-Geral de Assuntos Farmacêuticos, Avenida Columbano Bordalo Pinheiro, 87 – 1000 Lisboa, Portugal.

Singapore

Document reviewed:

SINGAPORE: A Guide on Drug Registration, Ministry of Health, Singapore. February 1987.

Address of Regulatory Agency:

Ministry of Health Singapore, 55 Cuppage Road, Cuppage Centre 09-00, Singapore 0922.

The relevant paragraphs are quoted in full below:

«5. Product licenses: 5.2.2. For new products the following information is needed:
- a) Full formula including inert ingredients.
- b) Detailed manufacturing procedure.
- c) Finished product specifications with certificate of analysis.
- d) Method of analysis of active ingredients.
- e) Registration Certificate/Certificate of Free Sale from the country of origin.
- f) Free sale certificates from other countries.
- g) Document from Health Authority of the country of origin certifying that the manufacturer concerned is a licensed pharmaceutical manufacturer.
- h) Specimen sales pack, label and pamphlet.
- i) Summary of the clinical trial papers on the product.

5.3. After a product has been licensed, any subsequent change in the particulars relating to the product (e.g. change of formula, composition/ingredients, recommended use) may render the licence invalid unless prior approval of such change has been obtained from the licensing authority.

5.4. Product holder should report to the Inspectorate Section, Ministry of Health, as soon as possible or within one week, any adverse drug reaction to the product.»

Note: The document does not contain specific requirements for toxicological studies.

Republic of South Korea

Documents reviewed:

REPUBLIC OF SOUTH KOREA I: Guidelines for the general toxicity test on drugs. NIH Guidelines no. 287, 1985.9.1

REPUBLIC OF SOUTH KOREA II: Guidelines for the special toxicity test on drug. NIH Guidelines no. 267, 1985,5.1

Address of Regulatory Agency:

Division Pharmaceutical Affairs, Bureau of Pharmacaeutical Affairs, Ministry of Public Health and Social Affairs. Chung Ang-Dong, Kwa Cheon-City, Shi Heung-Kun, Gyung Gi-Do. Republic of Korea 171.

Summary of Toxicological Guidelines:

REPUBLIC OF SOUTH KOREA I: Guidelines for the general toxicity test on drugs. NIH Guidelines no. 287, 1985 9.1

General

Experimental animals: Disease free animals of certified strains.

Acute toxicity or single dose effects

Species:	At least 2, one non-rodent if necessary.
Sex:	M and F.
Number of animals:	5 groups per sex. At least 5 and 2 animals per group for rodents and non-rodents respectively.
Route:	Orally or parenterally. Additionally, routes used in human application if necessary.
Dose levels:	More than 5.
Administration:	Once.
Observation period:	More than 2 weeks if administered orally, at least one week for s.c., i.v. or i.p. administration.
Determination of LD50:	Required.
Variables:	Toxic signs, body weight (measured at least 3 times), gross examination of autopsied animals at the end of observation period, histopathology of dead animals during experiment.

Subacute toxicity

Species:	At least 2, one non-rodent if necessary.
Sex:	M and F.
Number of animals:	At least 4 groups per sex, including control. At least 10 and 2 animals per group, for rodents and non-rodents respectively.

Administration:	Once a day, six times per week.
Dose levels:	More than 3, logarithmically decreased by equal ratio from LD10.
Route:	According to human application.
Duration:	Drugs to be administered in clinic once or for 1 to 4 weeks: 1 month. Drugs to be administerd in clinic for 1 week or less or for more than 4 weeks: 3 months.
Experimental procedure:	At least 10 animals of rodents and 2 of non-rodents of the lowest dose group should survive.
Variables:	Measurement of body weight, food intake and water consumption every two weeks. – Where necessary following tests should be performed on blood samples collected at autopsy and with urine samples collected at 1 week before autopsy: – Blood: protein, urea nitrogen, blood sugar, cholesterol, transaminases, alkaline phosphatase, sodium, potassium, chloride, bilirubin, and creatine, etc. RBC counts, WBC counts, WBC percentage, hemoglobin contents, hematocrit value, blood clotting time. – Urine: urine volume, pH, sugar, protein, hematuria, cast (precipitation). Weights of following organs: kidney, liver, spleen, heart, lung, thyroid gland, adrenal gland, brain, testis and ovary. Histopathology of above organs, bone marrow, and peripheral blood. Determination of maximum tolerated and harmless dose.

Chronic toxicity

Species:	At least 2.
Sex:	M and F.
Number of animals:	At least 4 groups per sex, including control.
Dose levels:	Maximum tolerated dose, intermediate dose, harmless dose.
Route:	According to human application.
Duration:	Drugs to be administered in clinic once or for 1 week or less: not required. Drugs to be administered in clinic for 1 to 4 weeks: 6 months. Drugs to be administered in clinic for more than 4 weeks: 1 year.
Experimental procedure:	At least 20 animals of rodents and 4 of non-rodents should survive at final observation.
Variables:	Measurement of body weight, food intake and water consumption every month. Where necessary, following tests should be performed on blood samples collected at autopsy and urine samples collected at 1 week before autopsy:

South Korea

- Blood: protein, urea nitrogen, blood sugar, cholesterol, transaminase, alkaline phosphatase, sodium, potassium, chloride, bilirubin, and creatine, etc. RBC counts, WBC counts, WBC percentage, hemoglobin contents, hematocrit value, blood clotting time.
- Urine: urine volume, pH, sugar, protein, hematuria, cast (precipitation).
Histopathology of animals which died during observation period.
Weights of following organs: kidney, liver, spleen, heart, lung, thyroid gland, adrenal gland, brain, testis, and ovary.
Histopathology of above organs, bone marrow and peripheral blood.
Clinical test results if necessary. Determination of maximum tolerated dose and harmless dose.

Supplement

In the absence of any specific guidelines, the above could be applied to chemical substances.

REPUBLIC OF SOUTH KOREA II: Guidelines for the special toxicity test on drug. NIH Guidelines no. 267. 1985.5.1

General

Experimental animals: SPF animals in barrier system animal houses.

Fertility test

Species:	At least one among rats, mice etc.
Sex:	M and F.
Number of animals:	In case of rats and mice more than 20 of each sex per group.
Dose levels:	More than 3, excluding controls. Highest dose should be maximum dose tolerated by dams.
Control groups:	Non-treated control group, placebo-treated and solvent-treated group.
Route:	In accordance with expected clinical route.
Administration period:	More than 60 days using 40 day old M rats, and 14 days before mating to early stage of organogenesis of almost all organs for F using sexually mature animals.
Experimental procedure:	A treated M and a treated F should be housed together and observed every morning for confirmation of successful copulation. Mating period between the same M and F should be about 2 weeks. If necessary, a treated F and a non-treated M may be housed together and observed every morning for confirmation of successful copulation. When results positive, all dams should be autopsied at expected end of gestation period.

South Korea

Variables:	Number of corpora lutea, successful pregnancies, dead fetuses. Gross examinations of organs and tissues of living fetuses. M and F which failed to copulate should be autopsied at appropriate time.

Teratology test

Species:	At least 2, rabbit plus rat or mouse.
Number of animals:	More than 30 pregnant F per group for rats and mice, more than 12 pregnant F for rabbits.
Dose levels:	More than 3, excluding controls. Highest dose should be maximum dose tolerated by dams.
Control groups:	Non-treated group, placebo-treated and solvent-treated group.
Route:	Expected clinical route.
Administration period:	Continuously from day 6 to 15 of gestation in mice, 7 to 17 in rats and 6 to 18 in rabbits.
Experimental procedure:	1-2 days before expected date of delivery, Caesarean section of 2/3 of dams. Remaining 1/3 of dams should be allowed to deliver litter.
Variables:	Number of fetuses, position of fetuses in uterus horns, number of corpora lutea, dead fetuses and resorptions, weight of fetuses and examination of external, visceral and skeletal abnormalitites.

Peri- and postnatal test

Species:	At least 1, mice, rats or rabbits.
Number of animals:	More than 20 pregnant F per group for rats and mice, more than 12 pregnant F for rabbits.
Dose levels:	More than 3, excluding controls. Highest dose should be maximum dose tolerated by dams.
Control groups:	Non-treated group, placebo-treated and solvent-treated groups.
Route:	In accordance with expected clinical route.
Administration period:	Continuously from last 1/3 of gestation to weaning: from day 15 of gestation to day 21 after delivery in mice, from day 17 of gestation to day 21 after delivery in rats, and from day 18 of gestation to day 30 after delivery in rabbits.
Experimental procedure:	All dams should be allowed to deliver and nurse their young and should be examined for abnormality on delivery.
Variables:	Gestation period, mortality and weight of newborns, external and skeletal abnormalities of dead fetuses, lactation by dams, nursing instinct. Examination of effects of drug or its metabolites on neonates through dams. Autopsies of all dams at the end of lactation. Examination of growth and development, including behavior, specific signs and reproduction capacity of newborns.

South Korea

Another long-term observation study on progenies, and examination of other litter progenies of treated dams if necessary.

Carcinogenicity

Species:	At least 2, mice, rats or hamsters, etc.
Sex:	M and F.
Number of animals:	More than 50 of each sex per group.
Dose levels:	More than 3, excluding controls. Highest dose should be maximum tolerated dose which animals can survive in long term. Lowest dose should be maximum therapeutic dose in human, or dose that produces a pharmacological effect in same animals. Intermediate dose should be geometric mean of highest and lowest dose.
Control groups:	Non-treated group, placebo-treated and solvent-treated groups.
Route:	As expected for clinial use. If p.o. for humans, test substance to be administered continuously in the diet or drinking water. If in diet, concentration of test substance should be less than 5 %.
Administration period:	7 days per week. In case of forced oral administration, more than 5 days per week.
Experimental detail:	From more than 24 to less than 30 months for rats, from more than 18 to less than 24 months for mice and hamsters. For mice and hamsters, mortality based on reasons other than tumors should be below 50 % when autopsied after 24 months' treatment. Examination 1 to 3 months after treatment. When cumulative death index of low dose or control groups reaches 75 %, remaining animals should be killed and the test terminated.
Experimental procedure:	Daily observation of general condition of all animals. Measurement of body weight once a week for 3 months, then once every 4 weeks till the end of test. Autopsies and macroscopic examination of all animals.
Variables:	At autopsy: peripheral blood RBC, WBC, blood smear samples. In case of anemia, hypertrophy of lymph nodes, enlargement of liver and spleen or where blood diseases are suspected, blood smear samples should be examined.

Except for those neoplastic lesions and lesions suspected as neoplasm which can be observed macroscopically, pathological examination of all the following organs and tissues should be conducted: skin, mammary glands, lymph nodes, salivary glands, sternum, vertebrae and femur, thymus, trachea, lung and bronchi, heart, thyroid and parathyroids, tongue, esophagus, small intestine, colon, pancreas, spleen,

South Korea

adrenals and suprarenal gland, bladder, testis, ovaries, accessory genital organ, eyeball, brain, pituitary gland, spinal cord etc.

Mutagenicity

I In vitro test

1. Gene mutation tests

1) Salmonella strains reversion test

Strains:	TA 1535, TA 1537, TA 98, TA 100 etc.
Concentration of test substance:	At least 5, excluding control groups. Highest concentration should produce antimicrobial effect or be within the limit of 100 mg/plate or maximum soluble concentration. Reasons for selection of concentrations should be given. Metabolic activation: Mutagenicity test should be conducted both in the presence and absence of a metabolic activation system (Rat liver homogenats S-9 fraction).
Control groups:	Solvent-treated controls as negative controls. Known mutagens as positive control groups.
Evaluation of results:	If number of reverse mutation colonies is twice that of negative control and dose-dependence is proved, test result is judged as «positive». Test result should be recorded as real colony numbers and reasons for judgement should be given.

2) E. coli strains reversion test

Strains:	3, such as WP2, WP2 uvrA, WP2 uvrA pkM 101.
Concentration of test substance:	At least 5, excluding control groups. Highest concentration should produce antimicrobial effect or be within the limit of 100 mg/plate or maximum soluble concentration. Reasons for selection of concentration should be given.
Control groups:	Known mutagens as positive controls.

3) Mutagenicity evaluation in cultured cells of mammals

Cells:	Mouse lymphadenoma L 5178Y cells, Chinese hamster CHO or V 79 cells etc.
Concentration of test substance:	Highest concentration should be cytotoxic, or in case of noncytotoxic test substance, maximum soluble concentration.
Metabolic activation:	Suitable metabolic activation system should be used concurrently.
Exposure time:	2 to 5 hours, depending on nature of cells and test substance.
Evaluation of results:	Numbers of mutant cell colonies and survival rate of cells. Number of mutant cells vs. number of surviving cells.

South Korea

2. Chromosome mutation in cultured mammalian cells

Cells:	Primary cultured or subcultured cell lines of human or other mammalian cells.
Concentration of test substance:	At least 3. Standard concentration to be cell division inhibition concentration. Further concentration to include concentrations both higher and lower than standard concentration. Reasons for selection of concentrations should be given.
Metabolic activation:	Suitable metabolic activation system should be used concurrently.
Treatment time:	According to the cell division cycle, but where S-9 mix is present, its toxicity prevents determination of treatment time limit prediction. Chromosome preparations should be made at appropriate time after treatment.
Control groups:	Untreated and solvent-treated controls as negative controls. Known chromosome mutation inducing substances as positive control.
Variables:	Numbers of chromosomes and incidence of abnormal structured cells should be included. Metaphase of mitosis features of more than 100 cells per concentration should be observed.
Evaluation of results:	Test result is «positive», in case of significant increase of incidence of cells with chromosomal abnormalities compared to negative controls, and when dose-dependence is proved. Incidence of cells with chromosomal aberrations, frequency of chromosomal aberrations per cell, types of abnormal cell and evaluation standards should be recorded.

II In vivo test

1. Micronucleus test in rodents

Species:	Mice or other rodents.
Sex:	M and F.
Number of animals:	Not less than 6 sexually mature animals of each sex per group.
Dose levels:	At least 3. Highest dose should be derived from 1/2 dose of LD50. Selection of doses should be explained.
Route:	P.o. or i.p. once, and if necessary continuously.
Control groups:	Untreated or solvent-treated controls as negative controls. Known micronucleogenic substances as positive controls.
Experimental procedure:	18-30 hours after treatment, sacrifice of test animals. Preparation of bone marrow smear samples of femur bones. Observation of incidence of micronuclei in 1000 polychromatic erythrocytes per dose. Concurrent calculation of ratios of polychromatic erythrocytes to normochromatic erythrocytes.

South Korea

Evaluation of results:	Test result «positive», if increase of incidence of micronucleated cells significant. Mean value between groups, standard deviation and results of statistical evaluation should be recorded.

2. Dominant lethality test in the rodents

Species:	Mice or other rodents.
Sex:	M and F.
Number of animals:	Not less than 15 sexually matured animals of each sex per group per week.
Dose levels:	At least 2 for M. Highest dose should be derived from preliminary test dose, by which 100 % of animals can survive for 30 days.
Route:	P.o. or i.p.
Administration period:	Should be one of: single treatment or treatments continuous for 5 days or 6 weeks.
Mating:	Between males and virgin females.
Mating period:	For single treatment and continuous 5 days treatment groups: 6 weeks after last treatment. For continuous 6 weeks treatment group: 1 week after last treatment.
Control groups:	Untreated or solvent-treated controls as negative controls. Known dominant lethality inducing substances as positive controls.
Experimental procedure:	Caesarean section of F at later stage of pregnancy.
Variables:	Number of implanted embryos, corpora lutea, living or dead fetuses, embryos etc.
Evaluation of results:	Calculation of dominant lethality in percent according to the following formula:

$$DL(\%) = 1 - \frac{\text{mean No of living fetuses per pregnant female animal in treated groups}}{\text{mean No. of living fetuses per pregnant female animal in negative controls}} \times 100$$

Result «positive», if number of living fetuses decreases significantly with concurrent increase in number of dead embryos and if dose-dependency is proved.

3. Sex-linked recessive lethality test in the Drosophila melanogaster.

Strains:	Male, female Muller-5 strain and, if necessary, other strains.
Route:	Orally. Exposure to gaseous substances also acceptable.
Concentration of test substance:	2 to 3, including permitted maximum concentration. DMSO as solvent not advisable.
Control groups:	Known mutagens such as EMS or DMN as positive controls. Where a laboratory has control data, this procedure may be omitted.

South Korea

Experimental procedure:	Treated field M strain should be mated with normal F strain. After mating between litter progeny, observation of incidence of F2 M field strain. A low incidence implies mutation of germ cells in parents' M strain (This is an abbreviated version of the standard procedure as described in the guidelines).

4. Cell genetic test in mammalian bone marrow cells (in vivo test).

Species:	Rats or other rodents.
Sex:	M and F.
Number of animals:	Not less than 5 per sex.
Route:	P.o., i.p. or other.
Administration period:	Once or continuously.
Dose levels:	At least 3. Highest dose should be a toxic dose derived from LD50 value.
Experimental procedures:	6, 12 and 24 hours after treatment, preparation of bone marrow smear samples.
Variables:	Observation of 50 cells per animal in metaphase. Record of incidence of chromosomal aberrations.

Local toxicity

1. Epicutaneous irritation test

Species:	Rabbits weighing 2.0 to 3.0 kg.
Number of animals:	Not less than 6.
Dose level:	0,5 ml or 0,5 g on intact or dekeratinized skin.
Test procedure:	After application of test substance a patch (6 cm^2) should be applied to treated skin for 24 hrs.
Control:	Untreated adjoining intact skin of test animal to serve as control.
Observation period:	At 24 and 72 hrs after application.
Evaluation of results:	Description of erithema (using evaluation form derived from the original Draize procedure).

2. Eye irritation test

Species:	Rabbits weighing 2.0 to 3.0 kg.
Number of animals:	9 per group.
Dose level:	0,1 ml.
Test procedure:	Test substance should be instilled into one eye of each test animal. 2 and 4 seconds after instillation, instilled eyes of 3 animals respectively should be washed with 20 ml of warm water.

South Korea

Control:	Instilled eyes of remaining animal should be left untreated as control.
Observation period:	24, 48, 72 hrs, 4 and 7 days after instillation.
Evaluation of results:	Description of edema (using evaluation form derived from the original Draize procedure).

Inhalation toxicity test

1. Acute inhalation toxicity test

Species:	Rabbits, rats or guinea pigs.
Number of animals:	Not less than 4.
Test procedure:	After inhalation and exposure for 30 seconds, air should be inhaled for 15 minutes. This procedure should be repeated continuously not less than 10 times at an interval of 30 minutes.
Variables:	Toxic signs, food intake, body weight and hematology.
Observation period:	4 days.
Evaluation of results:	After observation period test animals should be sacrificed for histopathological examination.

2. Subactue inhalation toxicity test

Species:	Rabbits, rats or guinea pigs.
Number of animals:	Not less than 5.
Test procedure:	Test substance should be inhaled twice per day for 30 seconds, not less than 5 days per week for 4-12 weeks.
Variables:	Toxic signs, food intake, body weight and hematology.
Evaluation of results:	After observation period animals should be sacrificed for histopathological examination.

Supplement

Where there are no specific guidelines for chemical substances, these guidelines may be applied.

Spain

Document reviewed:

SPAIN: Ministerio de la Gobernacion. Decreto 1416/1973 sobre regulacion del Registro Farmaceutico. May 10, 1978.

Address of Regulatory Agency:

Direccion General de Farmacia y Productos Sanitarios, Ministerio de Sanidad y Consumo, Paseo del Prado, 18-20, 28014 Madrid, Espana.

In the above document no details of toxicity testing are given. The relevant paragraphs concerning registration of a pharmaceutical product are summarized below in English translation:

«Article 3, 1) and 2): A list of data and specifications of a drug and its active ingredients shall be submitted. The data must include: name (and international name) of drug, complete quantitative composition, fundamental therapeutic indications and other indications, studies of pharmacological action, pharmacodynamic, pharmacokinetic and toxicity studies, clinical trials, indication of usual therapeutic dose including minimum and maximum dose per day, clinical indications, contraindications, incompatibility and side effects, route of administration and justification of pharmaceutical form, blood and other body fluid levels, bibliography.» etc.

The following official documents regulating certain aspects of drug registration were reviewed:

– Decreto 2464/1963, de 10 de agosto. Laboratorios de especialidades farmacéuticas, registro, distribucion y publicidad (B.O.E. de 7 de octubre).
– Real Decreto 2730/1981 de 19 de octubre, sobre caracteristicas y registro de las especialidades farmacéuticas publicitarias (B.O.E. de 25 de noviembre).
– Orden de 17 de septiembre de 1982, de desarrollo del Real Decreto anterior (B.O.E. de 29 de septiembre).
– Orden de 16 de julio de 1986, por la que se modifica el contenido del Anexo de la Orden de 17 septiembre de 1982 (B.O.E. de 30 de julio).
– Real Decreto 944/1978, de 14 de abril, por el que se regulan los ensayos clinicos de productos farmacéuticos y preparados medicinales (B.O.E. de 6 de mayo).
– Orden de 3 de agosto de 1982, por la que se desarrolla el Real Decreto anterior (B.O.E. de 12 de agosto).

None contain additional requirements for toxicological studies.

Sri Lanka

Document reviewed:

SRI LANKA: The Gazette of the Democratic Socialist Republic of Sri Lanka, Extraordinary, No. 378/3, December 2, 1985. Regulations made by the Minister of Health, under section 38 of the Cosmetics, Devices and Drugs Act No. 27 of 1980 as amended by Act No. 38 of 1984 and approved by Parliament.

Address of Regulatory Agency:

Department of Health Sri Lanka, Formulary Committee Office, P.O. Box 271, Colombo, Sri Lanka.

Note:

To our knowledge, no new drugs are being developed in Sri Lanka.

The relevant paragraphs of the above regulations are cited below:

«Part I: Registration of Drugs:

4. ...the Authority shall prepare a register of every registered drug and shall enter or cause to be entered therein the following particulars relating to such registered drugs:
   a) the approved official name and brand name of the drug;
   b) the name of the manufacturer;
   c) the country of manufacture;
   d) the registration number assigned to it;
   e) the name and address of the holder of the Certificate of Registration;
   f) whether he is an importer or manufacturer; and
   g) the number of the licence issued to him.

Part III: Licence to Manufacture Drugs:

30. (2) No drug other than a registered drug ... shall be manufactured in Sri Lanka.

38. The Authority shall keep a register of every licensed manufacturer of drugs, and shall enter or cause to be entered therein the following particulars relating to each such licensed manufacturer:
   a) the name of such licensed manufacturer;
   b) the address of the premises at which he is authorised to manufacture the drugs in respect of which the licence has been issued;
   c) the number of the licence;
   d) the date of issue of the licence; and
   e) the number and date of the Certificate of Registration if issued to him under the Business Names Ordinance.

Schedule IV: Information Required for Registration of a Drug:

Applicant: Name, address, and status of applicant.

Sri Lanka

Drug: Name (brand name and official or approved name) and dosage form of the drug (e.g. tablet, syrup, injection).

Composition: Ingredients should be listed by their official or approved names and should include their exact quantities as per unit dose or if not practicable as percentage of their total formulation.

– Main pharmacological group (e.g. diuretic etc.).

*– A certificate from the health authorities of the country in which it is produced, confirming that the drug is in use there and the period of use and if not, reasons for not marketing it in the country of origin.

– Certificate of analysis and full information concerning analytical assay and other control methods to ensure identity, strength, quality and stability.

*– Published reports of controlled clinical trials, establishing therapeutic efficacy of drug. In the case of drug combinations, evidence must be provided to justify inclusion of all the active constituents in the formulation.

*– Summary of toxicity tests and tests for teratogenicity indicating safety of the drug.

– Data sheet giving following information:

a) Pharmacology: Pharmacological actions, mechanism of action (if known), relevant pharmacokinetic data.

b) – Clinical information: Indications, contraindications, precautions, warnings, adverse effects, drug interactions, dosage regimen, average dose and dose range for adults and children, dosing interval, average duration of treatment, dosage in special situations e.g. renal, hepatic and cardiac insufficiency.

– Overdosage: Brief clinical description of symptoms, treatment of overdosage.

c) Pharmaceutical information: Dosage forms and strengths of different dosage forms. Storage conditions and shelf life, package sizes, description of product e.g. tablet size, colour, markings etc.

*– List of countries in which drug is approved or registered for sale.

*– Fully packed samples of drug in form that will be offered for sale should also be sent, to enable analysis of product.

– Sample of label(s) used on containers should be supplied.

– All data should be submitted in English, in a hard file cover, in duplicate.

– Information marked with asterisk* is not required in case of drugs that have been already approved for import or local manufacture. In case of drugs approved for import, names should be in the Government gazettes published on July 18, 1980 and thereafter.»

Suriname

Note:

Being a developing country, neither new drugs nor diagnostics undergo preclinical or clinical safety testing in SURINAME. Specific rules and guidelines are therefore not available (letter from the Inspector of Health, November 30, 1987).

Address of Regulatory Agency:

Geneesmiddelen Registratie Commissie, Hoek Kernkampweg / A. Samsonstraat, Paramaribo, Suriname.

Sweden

Note:

SWEDEN uses the **Nordic Guidelines**.

Adress of Regulatory Agency:

Socialstyrelsen läkemedelsavdelning, Box 607, S-751 25 Uppsala, Sweden.

Switzerland

Document reviewed:

SWITZERLAND: Intercantonal Office for the Control for Medicaments (IOCM). Guidelines of the IOCM Concerning Documentary Requirements for the Registration of Medicaments for Use in Humans (Registration Guidelines). December 16, 1977, revised May 23, 1985.

Address of Regulatory Agency:

Interkantonale Kontrollstellle für Heilmittel, IKS, Erlachstrasse 8, CH-3012 Bern

Summary of Toxicological Guidelines:

Acute toxicity (single administration)

Species:	Use of primitive species or alternative methods whenever practicable. At least 2 experiments.
Sex:	Equal numbers of M and F.
Route:	At least 2 (p.o. and parenteral), including route proposed for use in man.
Observation period:	At least one week.
Determination of LD:	Only approximate LD50 required.
Variables:	E.g. hematological, biochemical, pathological and histopathological data.

Chronic toxicity (repeated administration)

Species:	At least 2 mammalian, rodent and non-rodent.
Duration:	At least 3 months. If substance will be used in man repeatedly, or for longer than a few weeks, duration to be 6 months, in certain cases 12 months or longer.
Route:	Route proposed for use in man (as far as practicable).
Dose levels:	Several times larger than that proposed for use in man. Highest dose must produce changes, however, most of animals must survive. Controls.
Variables:	Food intake, weight changes, growth, general behavior, hematology, organ functions, autopsy, histology.

Embryotoxic and teratogenic effects

Method:	Investigation of effect on fetus, possible effect on male or female fertility.
Procedure:	Not specified.

Switzerland

Carcinogenicity and mutagenicity

Requirement:
– When results from other investigations imply possible carcinogenic or mutagenic effects.
– When carcinogenic or mutagenic effect possible on the basis of pharmacological or biochemical properties.
– When drugs having similar chemical properties exhibit carcinogenic and mutagenic effects.

Fixed combinations

General requirement: Data on toxicological profile of combination and its components must be presented. In addition, whenever technically possible, information on absorption, distribution, biotransformation and excretion of components when administered in combination should be provided.

Topically administered drugs

General requirement: Local tolerance to single and repeated administration and determination of sensitizing properties in animals and man.

Histology: In animal experiments the application sites must be examined histologically.

Pharmacokinetics: When technically possible absorption should be determined.

Systemic toxicity: Necessary when significant absorption of topically administered drug observed.

Taiwan

Document reviewed:

TAIWAN: The Regulations for Applying Drug Registration in Taiwan. February 25, 1981.

Address of Regulatory Agency:

National Health Administration. Taiwan, R.O.C.

This document contains rules and regulations for registration of drugs in Taiwan. It gives no guidelines about toxicity testing, but states that toxicity tests must be performed for the following categories of drugs:

    1. New drugs not yet included in pharmacopeia:
        A) New structures
        B) Existing and approved drugs but with different presentation (formulation)
        C) Existing and approved drugs but different in administration

Requirement: Acute, subacute, chronic toxicity and teratogenicity

    2. Combinations of more than 3 approved drugs
        A) Different from existing combinations (ingredients and quantities)

Requirement: Acute, subacute and chronic toxicity

No toxicology required for   B) Containing same approved drugs as existing combination, but different daily dosage, administration and indications

Note: This regulation also describes extent of clinical trials.

Thailand

Document reviewed:

THAILAND: Letter from the Deputy Secretary-General of the Food and Drug Administration of Thailand, September 23, 1987.

Address of Regulatory Agency:

Drug Control Division, Food and Drug Administration, Ministry of Public Health, Devaves Palace, Samsen Rd., Bangkok 10200, Thailand

Note:

Thailand has no specific guidelines, however for preclinical safety testing of new drugs and diagnostics prior to clinical investigation full toxicological and pharmacological evaluation is required and the results must be approved by the Thai FDA.

Details of drug registration procedures are described in :«National Drug Use and Control» by Pakdee Pothisiri, Ph.D., Food and Drug Administraion, Thailand, December 5, 1986.

Trinidad

Document reviewed:

TRINIDAD: Ministry of Health and Environment. Food and Drugs (Amendment) Regulations, 1969.

Address of Regulatory Agency:

Chemistry/Food and Drugs Division, 115, Frederick Street, Port of Spain, Trinidad, West Indies.

In the above document no details of toxicity testing are given. The relevant paragraphs concerning the manufacture and import of drugs are reproduced below:

«Division 3 – New Drugs.

...

2. No person shall import, sell or advertise for sale a new drug unless he has been granted permission in accordance with paragraph 12 or unless

    a) the manufacturer or importer has filed with the Minister in duplicate a new drug submission in respect of that drug; and

    b) the Minister has issued a notice of approval in respect of the new drug to the manufacturer or importer and such approval has not been withdrawn in accordance with paragraph 8.

3. Subject to paragraph 4, a new drug submission in respect of a drug to be imported shall contain:

    a) a description of the new drug ... and a declaration of the proper name, if any, and the name under which it is proposed to be sold;

    b) a statement of all the ingredients, the route of administration, the proposed dosage, the claims to be made for the new drug, the contraindications and side-effects of the new drug if known, and a description of the pharmaceutical form under which the new drug is to be sold;

    c) details of the tests applied to control the potency, purity and safety of the new drug;

    d) a draft of every label proposed to be used in connection with the drug;

    e) samples of the new drug in the finished pharmaceutical form in which it is to be sold; and

    f) such samples of the components of the new drug as the Director may require, and shall include one or more of the following; ...

    h) a certificate from the FDA of the Dept. of Health, Education and Welfare of the USA certifying that the new drug is

Trinidad

approved for use in the USA under the conditions of use recommended and giving the conditions under which it may be sold in the USA;
i) a certificate from the Ministry of Health of the UK ...
j) a certificate from the Dept. of Health of Australia ... or
k) a certificate in the English language, respecting the safety of the new drug for conditions of use recommended and giving the conditions under which it may be sold, issued by an official body or Government Dept. having authority to issue such certificate, such official body or Government Dept. having experience and facilities for testing the safety of new drugs that are considered by the Minister as adequate to ensure the safety of the new drug under the conditions of use recommended;

but the Minister may accept a submission made in accordance with paragraph 4.

4. The Minister may in his discretion accept a new drug submission that contains information specified in subparagraphs a-f of paragraph 3, and that includes:
a) detailed reports of the tests made to establish the safety of the new drug for the purpose and under the conditions of use for which it is recommended; ...

5. ... no person shall import, sell or advertise for sale a new drug in respect of which notice of approval has been given if any material change has been made in
a) the conditions of use of the drug, including the indications for use and the route of administration
b) its labels
c) the pharmaceutical form in which it is sold
d) the dosage of the new drug; or
e) the strength, purity or quality of the drug;

which is significantly different from the information contained in the new drug submission filed in respect thereof unless the manufacturer or importer has filed in duplicate with the Minister a supplement to the new drug submission that is satisfactory to the Minister and that describes the changes and gives all the particulars respecting the safety of the new drug and the revised conditions contained in the supplement.

6. Where notice of approval in respect of a new drug has been issued to a manufacturer or importer, another manufacturer or importer of the same new drug may provide the Minister with a submission that satifies the provisions of paragraph 4. ...

Division 8 – Conditions, facilities and controls for drug manufacture
...
2. No drug manufacturer shall sell a drug in the finished pharmaceutical form in which it is sold to the general public unless the drug has been manufactured, preserved, stored, labelled and tested under suitable conditions as provided in this

Trinidad

Division, and a Certificate to this effect has been issued by the Director, on the advice of the Drug Advisory Committee.

3. For the purposes of paragraph 2 of this Division, suitable conditions in respect of a drug requires: ...

    k) that records shall be kept in form, manner and content satisfactory to the Director showing
        i) for each batch or lot of the drug
            aa) the tests on the raw or bulk material used in manufacturing;
            bb) the tests on the drug in finished pharmaceutical form; ...
        ii) details of the manufacturing process, tests, procedures, and known hazards and stability of the drug

...

7. A drug manufacturer in a country other than Trinidad and Tobago shall be deemed to have complied with paragraphs ..., if the manufacturer or importer of a drug or drugs has produced to the Director a certificate concerning the sale, safety, or manufacture of the drug or drugs issued by

    a) the Dept. of National Health and Welfare of Canada
    b) the Dept. of Health, Education and Welfare of the US, or a State or City authority in the US concerned with health or pharmacy
    c) the Ministry of Health of the UK
    d) the Dept. of Health of Australia
    e) any Government Dept. or official body in other countries issuing such certificates as comply with Regulation 10 or paragraph 3 k) of Division 3 of this Schedule, which are considered by the Director to show that adequate standards for conditions of drug manufacture are enforced in those countries in respect of that drug manufacturer. ...»

Turkey

Document reviewed:

TURKEY: Ministry of Health and Social Assistance, Directorate of Pharmaceuticals: Ministerial Provisions Concerning to Turkish Pharmaceuticals. Ankara, 1986.

Address of Regulatory Agency:

Directorate-General of Pharmaceuticals, Ministry of Health & Social Assistance, Mithat Pasa Cad., Ankara, Sihhiye, Turkey.

Note:

No new drugs are being developed in Turkey, therefore, there are no guidelines to regulate preclinical safety studies. However, for new drugs already registered in other countries the manufacturer or importer must provide all information on safety studies and tests performed by the original manufacturer. The relevant paragraphs of the above document are copied (verbatim) below:

«**Part 7.** Regulation concerning the importation of drug materials, starting materials, pharmaceuticals and medical preparations.

Drug Specifications: **Article 5:** The specifications for medicines to be imported are the same as the registered specifications in the Country of Origin and must be approved by the Ministry.

Certification of Starting Material Producers: **Article 6:** A document to be issued by the health authority of the starting material exporting country authenticating that the starting material has been produced according to the proper specifications, is requested.
etc.

Part 11. Registration Procedures.
VII. New Drug Registration Requirement.

1. Procedure for Samples:
a) All necessary documents are to be submitted to commission. When the registration is approved, the corporation is informed accordingly and import permission in sufficient quantities for raw material which cannot be obtained at market, is issued, to enable the corporation to submit samples.
b) Conditions outlined in paragraph a) are to be complied with and registration done for drugs proving satisfaction in their analysis. Permission for subject drugs' manufacture and sales will also be granted. Long-term stability studies are to be undertaken by the corporation.

Turkey

VIII. Application Procedures for Drugs to be Imported.

1. Complete information requested in Part 1 for drugs that will be manufactured in this country and that contain active substances which will enter into Turkey for the first time.
2. Agreement by the Main Factories indicating approval of importation.
3. Original printed prospectus.
4. Original formula.
5. The originals of free sales certificates for the drug as ratified by Main Factory, local Turkish Consulate and Health Authorities and Turkish translation of these documents in Public Notary approved copies.» etc.

United Kingdom (UK)

Note:

UK uses the **EEC Guidelines** and **UK Guidelines**.

Document reviewed:

UK: Department of Health and Social Security: Medicines Act 1968. Guidance Notes on Applications for Product Licences (MAL 2), revised December 1985, first published 1986.

Address of Regulatory Agency:

Department of Health and Social Security, Market Towers, 1 Nine Elms Lane, London SW8 5NQ.

Summary of Toxicological Guidelines:

Acute toxicity

Scope of study:	To give indication of likely effects and acute overdosage in man and information for the design of repeated dose toxicity and reproduction studies on relevant species.
Species:	At least 2 mammalian of known strain, unless use of a single species can be justified.
Sex:	Equal numbers of M and F. If no difference in response is observed between M and F of the first rodent species, then only one sex must be used in the other studies.
Route:	2, one identical with or similar to that proposed for use in man, the other ensuring systemic absorption of substance. If route proposed for use in man is i.v., this route alone is acceptable.
Observation period:	To be fixed by investigator as being adequate to reveal tissue or organ damage or recovery, usually 14 days, not less than 7 days, but without exposing animals to prolonged suffering.
Determination of LD50:	Quantitative evaluation of LD and information on dose effect relationship, but high level of precision is not required.
Method:	To be designed to obtain maximal relevant information from smallest possible number of animals.
Autopsy:	All animals.
Variables:	Signs observed including local reactions. Histopathology of any organ showing macroscopic changes at autopsy.

Toxicity with repeated administration

Species:	At least 2 mammalian, one a non-rodent. Species selected should metabolise the drug as similar to man as possible.

UK

	Agent should demonstrate pharmacological activity in species and strain used. No albino animals for toxicological evaluation of drugs that demonstrate melanin binding.
Sex:	Normally equal numbers of M and F.
Duration:	To be determined by proposed duration of usage in man and by pharmacokinetics of compound.

Intended duration of dosing in man	Duration of chronic toxicity tests in animals
– 1 or several doses on 1 day	14 days
– repeated, up to 7 days	28 days
– repeated, up to 30 days	90 days
– repeated, more than 30 days	180 days

Route:	As proposed for use in man. If different route used, reason for this to be discussed. I.p. not recommended, unless proposed as clinical route. Quantity of drug absorbed from proposed site of administration should be known from pharmacocinetic studies.
Dose levels:	3.
	– Highest dose to cause target organ toxicity.
	– Lowest dose should relate to proposed therapeutic dose.
	– Intermediate dose(s) should be spaced geometrically.
Number of animals:	Treatment groups large enough to:
	– reveal all toxicologically important effects due to treatment
	– allow sacrifice of animals at intervals before end of study
	– retain some animals for reversibility study.
Control groups:	To be included in all studies.
Frequency of administr.:	7 days per week. When rate of elimination is slow, less frequent. When rate of elimination is rapid, more than once a day.
Variables:	Food consumption, body weight, behavior and condition of the animals, hematology, biochemistry, urinalysis, ophthalmology monitoring (desirable). Histopathology of all organs from high-dose animals and controls, and of any tissues from any animals in any groups in which macroscopic lesions are found at autopsy.
	Tissues to be studied histologically:
	Gross lesions, tissue masses or tumors, blood smears, lymph nodes, mammary glands, salivary glands, sternebrae, femur or vertebrae, pituitary, thymus, trachea, lungs, heart, thyroid, esophagus, stomach, small intestine, colon, liver, gallbladder, pancreas, spleen, kidneys, adrenals, bladder, prostate, testes, ovaries, uterus, brain, eyes, spinal cord.
Immunotoxicology:	Selection of techniques used and choice of other tests appropriate to current state of knowledge and to species used.
Autopsy:	All animals.

UK

Toxicity tests for agents to be administered by special routes

Requirements:	Where proposed clinical route includes i.v., i.m., intra-arterial, intradermal, or s.c. administration, toxicology of appropriate duration with respect to proposed clinical usage should be conducted by these routes.
	Attention should be paid to injection sites with respect to any local reaction.

Intraperitoneal:
Unless proposed clinical route is by this route, use of i.p. route for repeated-dose studies is not recommended.

Inhalation:

Species:	2.
Dosing:	Frequency and duration of dosing determined by intended clinical use.
Control groups:	Additional control group for propellant or dispersing agent alone.
Procedure:	Studies should be performed using proposed clinical formulation with respect of drug plus propellant system or drug plus dispersing agent. A novel propellant should be investigated to same standard as a new active substance. Whole-body exposure should normally be avoided.
	Effectiveness of dosing must be established and attempts should be made to measure blood level of drug and, where appropriate, propellant. Estimate of amount of drug trapped on turbinates, in mouth, swallowed and that reaching lower respiratory tract is desirable.
Metabolic pattern:	It should be determined whether there are any pharmacokinetic or metabolic differences of relevance to the interpretation of toxicological studies conducted by inhalation route.
Local effects:	Respiratory tract should be studied with respect to ciliary activity and mucus secretion following both single and repeated exposure.
Variables:	Systemic effects should be studies with respect to serial observation, hematological, biochemical monitoring etc.
Autopsy:	Weight of lungs of all animals and histopathological examination of tissues taken from all exposed levels of respiratory tract and from associated lymphoid tissue.

Topical
a) Cutaneous

Species:	2.
Dosing:	Duration and frequency of dosing per day, determined by intended clinical use.

UK

Procedure:	Formulation intended for clinical use should be used. Whether studies on both intact and damaged skin are desirable depends on clinical use of drug. It is essential to clean treated area before applying subsequent doses.
Variables:	Percutaneous absorption should be measured and systemic and local effects should be monitored. Serial hematological and biochemical monitoring should be conducted on adequate number of animals from each dosed group. Autopsy of all animals.
Note:	If absorption is negligible, reproduction studies may be omitted provided that data are presented which demonstrate that appreciable amounts of drug are not systemically available.

b) Ophthalmic preparations

Requirements:	Tests for local toxicity are required for all ophthalmic preparations.
Dosing:	Duration and frequency of dosing determined by proposed clinical use.
Note:	Systemic effects following absorption should be considered for new chemical entities following ophthalmic administration.

c) Other routes

Appropriate studies should be conducted for these routes, e.g. aural, nasal, rectal, intravaginal etc.

Fetal toxicity and fertility studies

Scope of study:	To reveal the presence of any drug effect on each of the following mechanisms: – Damage to M and F gametes resulting in sterility or in production of abnormal young – embryogenesis – toxic effects on fetus – maternal metabolism producing secondary effects on fetus – effects on uterine growth or development – on parturition – on post-natal development and suckling of progeny and on maternal lactation – late effects on progeny.
Species:	– Teratogenicity studies: 2 mammalian, one a non-rodent. – Fertility and pre- and post-natal studies: 1.
Dose levels:	3. – Highest dose to produce some maternal toxicity, e.g. 10 % reduction in body weight gain. – Lowest dose to produce a pharmacodynamic effect similar

	to desired therapeutic effect, or to produce blood levels comparable to those required to produce the effect.
	– Intermediate dose: geometric mean of high and low doses.
Control groups:	In all studies.
Route:	As proposed for use in man, where practicable.
Duration:	– Teratogenicity studies: throughout period of embryogenesis
	– Fertility study: dosing on M and F at sufficient time before proposed mating to reveal any effect of drug on gametogenesis. F should be dosed throughout pregnancy.
	– Pre- and post-natal studies: throughout period of gestation from end of organogenesis to parturition and throughout period of lactation up to weaning.
Number of animals:	Adequate number of animals at each dose level to enable valid assessments to be made:
	– Teratogenicity studies: a minimum of 20 pregnant F rodents or 12 pregnant F non-rodents per dose.
	– Pre- and post-natal studies: 12 dams per dose.
	– Fertiliy studies: 24 dams per dose.
Experimental procedure:	Fertility study: dosed animals to be mated with dosed partners but in event of positive findings of a reproductive defect, study to be repeated using dosed animals mated with undosed partners. After mating half of F to be killed during gestation, some days before expected date of parturition, and fetuses to be removed by Caesarean section. The remainder of the F should be allowed to litter normally and rear their progeny. A large enough number of progeny should be allowed to live and reach maturity. Late effects on progeny in terms of auditory, visual and behavioral function should be assessed. Reproductive function to be determined in progeny by allowing one M and one F from each litter of dosed animals to breed and produce one litter (no brother/sister mating).
Variables:	– Teratogenicity studies: number of implantation sites and resorptions, weight and sex of individual fetuses. Examination of individual fetuses for external, skeletal and/or visceral abnormalities.
	– Fertility study: number of corpora lutea, rest as above.
	– Pre- and post-natal studies: animals killed at the end of lactation should be autopsied. Some of progeny may be allowed to live and reach maturity so that their reproductive capacity can be assessed. Other late effects on progeny (e.g. behavioral, visual and auditory function) should be determined.

UK

Carcinogenicity

Requirement:	Where substance would be used in man continuously for long periods (more than 6 months) or have a frequent intermittent usage.
	Where substance has a chemical structure that suggests carcinogenic potential.
	Where a substance causes concern as a result of:
	– some specific aspects of its biological action
	– its pattern of toxicity of long-term retention detected in previous studies
	– the findings in mutagenicity tests and/or short-term carcinogenicity tests.
Species and strain:	2, selection of species to be made on the basis of metabolic similarity to man. The responses of known species and strains to similar chemicals should be taken into account. No species with high or variable incidence of spontaneous tumor formation. Rat (outbred) and mouse (Fl hybrid) or known strain of hamster (outbred) with low incidence of neoplasm and good longevity recommended.
Dose levels:	3.
	– Highest dose to produce a minor toxic effect, e.g. 10 % weight reduction, or minimal target-organ toxicity.
	– Lowest dose should be of the order of 2-3 times the maximum daily therapeutic dose or dose that produces pharmacological effect in animals.
	– Intermediate dose: geometric mean of high and low doses. Exception: where toxic dose of drug is a high multiple of therapeutic dose it is acceptable if highest dose is set at 100 times the therapeutic dose.
Route:	As proposed for clinical use where possible. Where relevant, evidence of absorption should be provided.
Frequency of administr.:	Daily.
Duration:	Start: as soon as possible after weaning.
	Rat for 24 months, mouse and hamster 18 months. Where malignancy of tumor is in doubt, rat 30 months, mouse 24 months.
Sex:	M and F.
Number of animals:	Mice, rats and hamsters: 50 per treatment group and sex.
Control groups:	100 animals of each sex dosed with the vehicle by the same route. Possibly 2 separate control groups of 50 animals per sex.
Animal husbandry:	Standard conditions in terms of diet, housing and handling.
Experimental procedure:	Study should be designed to obtain maximum amount of information from animals used. Details of absorption, distri-

UK

	bution and metabolism of drug, and whether drug accumulated or was an enzyme inducer, should have been determined during intermediate-term toxicity studies.
Variables:	During study: animals should be regularly observed for general health and examined clinically to determine incidence and time of appearance of tumors. Food consumption and body weight should be recorded at regular intervals. Final investigations: microscopic examination of all tissues and organs from all high dose animals and all controls, as well as from middle and low-dose groups when necessary. Histopathology of same organs and tissues as in repeated administration (p 158).
Evaluation:	Statistical procedure used should be clearly stated. Data required: total incidence of tumor bearing animals and of tumors. Incidence of benign/malignant tumors involving a specific tissue. Time to tumor recognition.
Interpretation of results:	Strongest evidence that a compound is a carcinogenic hazard for man is epidemiological, although most known human carcinogens are found to be carcinogenic for experimental animals. There is no evidence that all substances which are carcinogenic for animals are also carcinogenic for man. Extrapolation to man is difficult: Criteria vary with agent under consideration, its projected use, dosage and mode of administration and also on species, sites, incidence of tumors and required test dosage.
Short-term studies:	Available techniques for short-term testing of chemicals for mutagenicity/transformation not at present capable of replacing formal carcinogenicity testing in animals. Short-term studies giving positive results will always indicate need for formal carcinogenicity studies, those giving negative results do not preclude need for formal studies.

Mutagenicity: see **EEC IV Guidelines**

USA

Documents reviewed:

USA I: Guideline for the Format and Content of the Nonclinical/Pharmacology/Toxicology Section of an Application. U.S. Department of Health and Human Services, Public Health Service, Food and Drug Administration. February 1987.
USA II: W. D'Aguanno. Drug Toxicity Evaluation – Preclinical Aspects. 1976.
USA III: W. D'Aguanno. Guidelines for Reproduction Studies for Safety Evaluation of Drugs for Human Use. 1976. (Based on: FDA Guidelines for Reproduction Studies for Safety Evaluation of Drugs for Human Use. January 1966).
USA IV: Guideline for the Format and Content of the Summary for New Drug and Antibiotic Applications. U.S. Department of Health and Human Services, Public Health Service, Food and Drug Administration. February 1987.
USA V: Federal Register, Part II, Department of Health and Human Services, Food and Drug Administration, New Drug and Antibiotic Regulations; Final Rule. February 22, 1985.
USA VI: Federal Register, Part VII, Department of Health and Human Services, Food and Drug Administration, New Drug, Antibiotic, and Biologic, Drug Product Regulations; Final Rule. March 19, 1987.
USA VII: Preface, Pharmaceutical Manufacturers Association (PMA), Guidelines for the Assessment of Drug and Medical Device Safety in Animals. February 1977.
USA VIII: Final Report to the Commissioner Food and Drug Administration, Agency Steering Committee on Animal Welfare Issues. U.S. Department of Health and Human Services, Public Health Service, Food and Drug Administration, August 15, 1984.

Addresses:

Center for Drugs and Biologics (CDB), Food and Drug Administration (FDA), Rockville MD 20857, U.S.A. (**USA I-IV**)
    (responsible for implementing drug investigations and marketing)
– CDB's Office of Biologics Research and Review (OBRR).
    (responsible for decisions on anti-infective, endocrine and metabolic drugs, vaccines and other biological products)
– CDB's Office of Drug Research and Review (ODRR)
    (responsible for review of other drug categories)
Center for Drugs and Biologics (HFN-362), Food and Drug Administration, 5600 Fishers Lane, Rockville, MD 20857, U.S.A. (**USA V**)
Dockets Management Branch (HFA-305), Food and Drug Administration, 5600 Fishers Lane, Rockville, MD 20857, U.S.A. (**USA VI**)
Pharmaceutical Manufacturers Association (PMA), 1155 Fifteenth Street, N.W. Washington, D.C. 20005, U.S.A. (**USA VII**)
U.S. Dept. of Health and Human Services, Public Health Service, FDA, Rockville, Maryland 20857, U.S.A. (**USA VIII**)

USA

USA I: Guideline for the Format and Content of the Nonclinical/Pharmacology/Toxicology Section of an Application. U.S. Department of Health and Human Services, Public Health Service, Food and Drug Administration. February 1987.

Summary of Toxicological Guidelines:

Note:

This document describes the format of a toxicological dossier and does not contain detailed protocol requirements.

Acute toxicity

Age of animals, route, vehicles, dose levels and volumes should be specified for each study.

Toxic signs, their onset, progression, or reversal should be described for each species. Mortality, time of death.

Lethal dose data (approximate or calculated median, limit doses, etc.) should be tabulated for interstudy and/or interspecies comparison.

For new FDA policy on acute toxicity testing see USA VIII.

Subchronic/chronic/carcinogenicity studies

Description of each study should include the following information: Species, strain, age, number of animals of each sex per group at beginning and end of study, dose levels, route, vehicle, control treatment, duration of treatment and of study, interim sacrifice, etc.

Within each study the following data should be presented: Observed effects, mortality, body weight, food/water consumption, physical examinations, hematology/bone marrow/coagulation, blood chemistry/urinalysis/ADME data, organ weights, gross pathology, histopathology.

Tumor data: Chronological list including period in which tumor was discovered, site and type of tumor, malignancy, and whether animal was sacrificed or died.

Reproduction studies

Studies should be presented in following sequence:
- Segment I – fertility and reproductive performance
- Segment II – teratology
- Segment III – perinatal-postnatal
- Other studies – multigeneration, etc.

Observations and their incidence should be presented in following order:
- Maternal effects and day of parturition/necropsy.
- Maternal necropsy: corpora lutea, uterine contents, implantations, dead fetuses.
- Fetuses: sex ratio, weight, viability, gross observations, visceral and skeletal abnormalities.
- Neonates to weaning: sex ratio, viability, growth, behavior and performance, anatomical abnormalities.

USA

Mutagenicity
Studies should be presented in following order:
  In vitro non-mammalian cell system
  In vitro mammalian cell system
  In vitro mammalian system
  In vivo non-mammalian system

Note:
Current FDA views on the role of mutagenicity studies in drug safety evaluation were presented by Vera C. Glocklin, Ph.D., of the FDA during a symposium entitled «Critical Evaluation of Mutagenicity Tests», February 22-25, 1982, in Berlin. (NMV, Mediziner-Verlag München, 1984). The relevant points of the FDA position can be summarized as follows:
«At the present time FDA does not require mutagenicity testing for human drugs or food additives.
Testing is occasionally recommended (a recommendation of FDA is an advisory opinion but not imposed regulatory obligation).
FDA usually recommends mutagenicity studies for certain categories of drugs such as antiviral, antipsoriatics and immunosuppressant agents.
If microbial assays are submitted and show positive or questionable results, it is recommended to use mammalian cell assays.
FDA has not yet attempted to develop a specific guideline for mutagenicity studies for drugs and has not endorsed any proposed guideline. For the few drug categories of particular concern FDA in general asks for information on microbial and mammalian cell mutagenicity test, chromosome effects, DNA repair and cell transformation, but test selection is generally left up to the applicant.»

USA

In 2 papers published by W. D'Aguanno, USA II and USA III, some specific recommendations are made. They are summarized below:

USA II: W. D'Aguanno. Drug Toxicity Evaluation – Preclinical Aspects. 1976.

Acute toxicity
(single dose treatment, or multiple dose over a period of 24 hrs. or less)

Determination of LD:	LD50.
Variables:	Motor activity, tremors, convulsions, loss of righting reflex, ataxia, sedation, ptosis, lacrimation, salivation, diarrhea, writhing; effects on respiration, depression, stimulation, blanching, cyanosis, vasodilatation, etc.
Note:	For new FDA policy on acute toxicity testing see USA VIII.

Subacute and subchronic toxicity

Duration:	2-4 weeks to 90 days.

Chronic toxicity

Species:	2, usually rat and dog. Occasionally a third species, e.g. monkey.
Duration:	For drugs given once or twice: 2 to 4 weeks. For clinical use of unlimited duration: 18 months for rat, 12 months for non-rodent species.
Administration:	Daily single dose; divided dose when acute dose is limited by drug effects. 7 days per week.
Route:	Same as proposed for use in man; usually p.o. In rodents administration as admixture to diet, if not practical by gavage.
Dose levels:	3: highest to produce some toxicity. Control group.
Variables:	Behavioral changes, general condition, food consumption, body weight.
	Periodically: ophthalmological examination. Hematological, biochemical and organ function tests. Autopsy, histopathology.

Toxicity studies on steroidal contraceptives

Prior to clinical Phase II:
Species:	Dog, monkey and rodent.
Duration:	At least one year.

Prior to clinical Phase III:
Species:	Dog, monkey and rat.
Duration:	Dog: up to 7 years must be under way
	Monkey: up to 10 years

USA

Note:	2-year-studies in rats, dogs and monkeys must be completed. WHO has proposed new toxicological guidelines for steroid contraceptives (see WHO pp 187). It is probable that these guidelines will be accepted by the US Food and Drug Administration.

Reproduction studies

Purpose: Determination of drug's potential effects on all aspects of reproductive process (fertility of M and F, conception, nidation, development and survival of embryo and fetus, parturition, lactation, viability and development of offspring and quality of mother's milk).

Methods: See USA III, below.

A more complete summary is given in the table reproduced below:

For animal toxicity studies

Category	Duration of Human Administration	Phase (1)	Subacute or Chronic Toxicity (2)
A. Oral	Several Days	I,II,III,NDA	2 species; 2 weeks
or parenteral	Up to 2 Weeks	I	2 species; 2 weeks
		II	2 species; up to 4 weeks
		III, NDA	2 species; up to 3 months
	Up to 3 Months	I, II	2 species; 4 weeks
		III	2 species; 3 months
		NDA	2 species; up to 6 months
	6 Months to unlimited	I, II	2 species; 3 months
		III	2 species; 6 months or longer
		NDA	2 species; 12 months or longer(N-r) 18 months (R)
B. Inhalation (General Anesthetics)		I,II,III,NDA	4 species; 5 days (3 hours/day)
C. Dermal	Single Application	I	1 species; single 24-hour exposure followed by 2-week observation
	Single or Short-term Appl.	II	1 species: 20-day repeated exposure (intact or abraded skin)
	Short-term Appl.	III	As above
	Unlimited Appl.	NDA	As above, but intact skin study extended up to 6 months

USA

D. Oph-thalmic	Single Appl.	I	
	Multiple Applications	I, II, III	1 species; 3 weeks daily applications as in clinical use
		NDA	1 species; duration commensurate with period of drug administr.
E. Vaginal or Rectal	Single Appl.	I	
	Multiple Applications	I, II, III, NDA	2 species; duration and number of applications determined by proposed use
F. Drug Combinations (3)		I	
		II, III, NDA	2 species; up to 3 months

(1) Phases I, II, and III are defined in Paragraph 130 0 of the New Drug Regulations.
(2) Acute toxicity should be determined in 3 to 4 species; subacute or chronic studies should be by route to be used clinically.
(3) where toxicity data are available on each drug individually.
(N-r) = Non-rodents; (R) = Rodents

	Category Observations	Special Studies
A.	Body Weights, Food Consumption, Behavior, Hemogram, Coagulation Tests, Liver and Kindney Function Test, Fasting Blood Sugar, Ophthalmic Examination, Metabolic Studies, Gross and Microscopic Examinations, Others as Appropriate.	For parenterally administerd drugs: Irritation studies, compatibility with blood where applicable.
D.		Eye irritation tests, graded doses
E.		Local and systematic toxicity after vaginal or rectal applications in 2 species.
F.		LD50 by appropriate route, compared to components run concurrently in 1 species.

USA

USA III: W. D'Aguanno. Guidelines for Reproduction Studies for Safety Evaluation of Drugs for Human Use. 1976. (Based on: FDA. Guidelines for Reproduction Studies for Safety Evaluation of Drugs for Human Use. January 1966).

Reproduction studies

General remarks

Route:	Several may be employed, preferably same as intended clinical route.
Dosage levels:	At least 2, high dosage should be subtoxic, lower dosage should take into account proposed therapeutic dose and should be some multiple of this. In cases where dosage used proved to be embryocidal additional studies with lower dosage should be performed, since it is possible that a nonembryotoxic level may produce anomalies. Negative and in special cases positive control groups should be included.
Number of animals:	Rats and mice: at least 20 pregnant F per test group. Rabbits: at least 10 pregnant F per test group.
Combinations:	– No reproduction studies for combination of 2 or more drugs, if the effect of each drug on reproduction is known. – Reproduction studies required, if 2 drugs are to be combined and either or both have been shown to affect adversely the reproduction process.
Special cases:	When drug given by dermal route is not absorbed systemically no reproduction studies necessary.

USA

USA IV: Guideline for the Format and Content of the Summary for New Drug and Antibiotic Applications. U.S. Department of Health and Human Services, Public Health Service, Food and Drug Administration. February 1987.

Purpose of this guideline:	To assist preparation by manufacturer of **summary** of a new drug application (see chapter II E: Summary format and content, nonclinical pharmacology and toxicology summary).

USA V: Federal Register, Part II, Department of Health and Human Services, Food and Drug Administration, New Drug and Antibiotic Regulations; Final Rule. February 22, 1985.

Nonclinical Pharmacology and Toxicology Section (paragraph 314.50(d)(2)):
A description of the following studies is required:
> Toxicological consequences of drug's intended clinical uses, including acute, subacute and chronic toxicity, carcinogenicity and toxicities related to the drug's particular mode of administration or conditions of use. Effects of absorption, distribution, metabolism and excretion of drug in animals on reproduction and fetal development.

USA VI: Federal Register, Part VII, Department of Health and Human Services, Food and Drug Administration, New Drug, Antibiotic, and Biologic, Drug Product Regulations; Final Rule. March 19, 1987.

Regulations governing the submission and review of investigational new drug applications (IND Rewrite): Pharmacology and Toxicology Information (paragraph 312.23(a)(8)):
The following information is required:
> Integrated summary of toxicological effects of drug in animals and in vitro. Depending on nature of the drug and phase of investigation, results of acute, subacute, and chronic toxicity tests, tests of effects on reproduction and developing fetus, any special toxicity test appropriate to the drug's particular mode of administration or conditions of use, and any in vitro studies must be included.

USA

USA VII: Pharmaceutical Manufacturers Association (PMA), Guideline for the Assessment of Drug and Medical Device Safety in Animals. February 1977.

Note:
These guidelines are not an official governmental document. However, they are widely followed in the USA and appear to be (tacitly) accepted by the FDA.

Acute toxicity

General remarks:	In case of non-rodent, a range finding study may produce more useful information and may be substituted for acute toxicity study.
Species:	At least 3, one a non-rodent, ideally including those predominating in pharmacological testing and those likely to be used in multidose toxicity and reproduction studies.
LD50:	For rodents: determined by a standard statistical method. For non-rodents: approximate determination.
Route:	LD50 should be determined by proposed human route and one other route.
Observation period:	At least 1 week, or longer if overt signs persist or delayed deaths occur.

Subacute and chronic toxicity studies

Species:	At least one rodent and one non-rodent.
Sex:	M and F.
Number of animals:	Sufficient number per group for valid estimation of incidence and frequency of toxic effects. Rodents: 10-25 of each sex per group; non-rodents: 2-3 of each sex per group. Group size shall also depend on toxicity-mortality findings of subacute studies, interim sacrifices, reversibility evaluation and assessment of other aspects of toxicology such as carcinogenesis.
Control groups:	Each study must include control groups at least as large as largest treatment group.
Dose levels:	Highest dose should cause obvious toxicity or at least some demonstrable pharmacological effects. Lowest dose should have no serious deleterious effect. One or more intermediate dose levels to allow determination of incipient toxicity and dose-response relationship.

USA

Duration: Recommended duration of animal studies to support the 3 phases of clinical testing are as follows:

Limit of Human Drug Usage	Phase of Clinical Study	Duration of Animal Toxicity Studies
1-3 days	I, II, III, NDA	2 weeks
Up to 4 weeks	I, II,	4 weeks
	III, NDA	13 weeks
Up to 3 months	I, II,	13 weeks
	III, NDA	26 weeks
3 months or longer	I, II,	13 weeks
	III,	26 weeks
	NDA	52 weeks or longer

(NDA = New Drug Application)

Chronic studies to be prolonged beyond 1 year if any toxic manifestations warrant further observations, or if general toxicity testing is integrated with other toxicological assessments such as carcinogenic potential.

Observation period: Sufficient to allow determination of reversitility or drug-withdrawal phenomena.

Variables: Clinical observations, hematology, clinical chemistry, biopsy, necropsy, histopathology and alteration of cellular structures by electron microscopy and other special techniques.

Skin toxicity
a) General remarks

Studies should be conducted on final product which has been chemically and physically characterized. The toxicological properties with respect to skin contact of stabilizers, emulsifiers, perfumes, colorants, solvents, etc. may differ considerably. Chemical interaction and shelf-life should also be considered.

In animal studies, clinical conditions should be simulated as nearly as possible, particularly when preparations are intended for repeated or prolonged application. If there is likelihood of use on babies and children, tests should be performed using neonatal animals.

Effects of drugs should be evaluated on both abraded and intact skin and potentiating effects of sunlight (photosensitization, etc.) on fluorescent agents should be evaluated.

b) Primary irritation

Gross signs of primary irritation are erythema, edema, exfoliation, eschar formation or necrosis and, in humans, vesiculation. For quantitation each of these effects may be rated from 1-5, or by any arbitrary system corresponding roughly to none, very slight, slight, moderate, severe, etc. Each effect or combination of effects may occur as a result of a single exposure of a few seconds or of repeated exposures over hours, days or weeks of repeated exposures. Abraded skin is likely to be more sensitive than intact, skin. An occlusive bandage may enhance the drug's toxic properties.

USA

Species:	Normally albino rabbit. Also guinea pig, subhuman primate and weanling pig.
Method:	Hair may be clipped or shaved from back or belly. Material may be applied to cotton patches subsequently taped to skin. Properly bandaged rabbits may be maintained in cages and permitted to eat and drink normally. Small amounts of material may be applied to inner surface of rabbit ear to simulate unconfined exposure conditions.

c) Sensitization

Some chemicals produce allergic, serous contact-type dermatitis. Such materials are absorbed through skin and probably alter protein in a manner which elicits an antigen-antibody reaction that may be later manifested by a local dermatitis at the point of secondary contact. 2 simple, reliable laboratory approaches to this problem are available: One employs guinea pigs, the other humans. If guinea pigs show strong positive reactions there is usually little justification for proceeding to humans. Guinea pigs may be made more sensitive by use of adjuvants. Negative results with guinea pig should be confirmed by human testing.

Repeated insult patch test is based on capacity of a chemical to sensitize an animal when applied repeatedly to same skin site. Systemic sensitization may then be determined by challenging the animal, after a 2-3 week rest period, with chemical at a skin site remote from insult series. Sensitization is manifested by a pink to red skin reaction at site of secondary contact. Important: Chemical or drug used for challenge must not produce primary irritation (erythema). If test substance is a primary irritant, it should be diluted to a concentration that does not produce erythema from a 24-hour contact. Challenge with the vehicle should be performed as control.

Insult series of doses (2 or 3 per week for 2-3 weeks) may be applied, preferably to clipped nape of neck either as open or closed patch or by intradermal injection. Challenge dose is usually applied to clipped flank. In case of potent allergens, skin reaction may become positive during insult period.

Phototoxic properties may be evaluated on rats, mice and rabbits, photoallergic effects on man.

d) Systemic injury

Acute studies:	May be conducted on rabbits by removing hair and fitting trunk with a cuff. Measured amounts of test material are applied under cuff at several dose levels to establish a toxic dose.
Subacute/chronic studies:	
Species:	Rabbits.
Sex:	M and F.
Method:	Animals should be fitted with collar or harness and conditioned for about 2 weeks. Fresh abrasions should be made periodically.

USA

Duration:	Usually not more than 90 days. Materials should be removed with warm water at the end of each 7-hour daily exposure period.
Dose level:	10-15 % of trunk surface should be covered with thin layer of test material calculated on basis of g per kg body weight per day.
Controls:	Both vehicle and untreated controls necessary.
Variables:	Signs of toxicity.
Conclusion:	In event of significant absorption or toxicity, oral subacute toxicity, teratology, reproduction, and mutagenic studies should be considered.
Extrapolation to man:	Appreciable differences between animal and human skin from standpoint of penetration. Generally animal skin more permeable than human skin. From penetration viewpoint, back skin of weanling pig closely resembles human forearm.

e) Acneform dermatitis

Chloracne are more likely to be associated with manufacturing process than with final product. However, acnegens could exist as trace impurities in drugs.

Species:	Rabbit (ear).
Dose level:	Small amounts, 0.1 ml.
Application period:	Daily on repeated dose basis for 3 to 5 weeks.
Variables:	Production of blackheads or comedos with subsequent hyperplasia of entire ear.

f) Neoplasia

Tumorgenic potential of active material per se, final product or of both should be evaluated.

Effects of drugs on the eye

2 categories: a) drugs applied locally either by accident or for therapeutic purposes; b) drugs administered systemically with the eye as a target tissue. These compounds should be evaluated for systemic toxicity as well as ophthalmic effects.

Species:	Monkeys and dogs rarely. Rabbits most widely used. However, limitations, e.g.: lesser lacrimation in response to irritants compared with monkeys and human beings, lower rate of blinking compared with other species, lack of a well-developed Bowman's membrane such as is present in man.
Methods:	Ophthalmoscopy, biomicroscopy with fluorescein staining of the cornea and tonometry where appropriate. Electroretinography of a separate group of animals should be considered.

USA

Note: Animals in the chronic toxicity studies are suitable subjects for observation of systemic ocular abnormalities.
Variables: Histological examination useful.

Effects of drugs on the ear

2 categories of ototoxic drugs: Antibiotics (e.g. aminoglycosides) and diuretics. Also other agents, such as the salicylates and quinine (and its derivatives).
Ototoxicity may be vestibular, cochlear or both. Since vestibular apparatus may be damaged before cochlea (or vice versa) it is important that means employed to detect ototoxicity assess damage to both organs.

Methods:

Methods for assessing inner ear damage in laboratory animals have included the following:

Cochlear	Vestibular
A. Clinical:	
1. Preyer Reflex	1. Clinical Observation and Physical Examination (e.g., Ataxia, Positional Nystagmus, Integrity of Labrinthine Righting Reflex)
2. Behavioral Audiometry	2. Special Function Tests: Postrotatory Nystagmus, Opticokinetic Nystagmus, Caloric Nystagmus
	3. Conditioned Behavior
B. Electrophysiological:	
1. Cochlear Microphonic Potentials	1. Electronystagmography
C. Morphological:	
1. Histology	1. Histology
2. Phase-Contrast Microscopic Examination of Fresh Cochlea	2. Electron Microscopy
3. ElectronMicroscopy	

Recommendations: All new chemical entities, suspect and non-suspect drugs, proposed for systemic and/or ototopical administration should be subjected to routine ototoxicity screening as part of the general toxicological work-up.
Species: Usually guinea pig, however, also rat and dog for routine testing of the functional integrity of the cochlea (Preyer reflex). Cat most sensitive species for the assessment of acquired vestibular deficit.
«Suspect» drugs: 1. Compounds related chemically or pharmacologically to known ototoxic agents.
2. Nephrotoxic agents. Although not all are ototoxic, most of the drugs known to be ototoxic are nephrotoxic as well.

USA

	3. Compounds showing evidence of ototoxic activity in routine tests. For drugs in this class, further and considerably more thorough testing is recommended.
Methods:	Several test methods: A combination of clinical examination for vestibular damage and microscopic examination of fresh cochlea by phase contrast microscopy are recommended for the testing of «suspect» compounds.
Controls:	A positive control which damages cochlea and/or vestibule of the species being used should be included.
Variables:	Histological examination of kidneys from affected animals may be helpful. Vestibular function (cats): Development of vestibular incoordination of body and head, postural deviation of head. Status of righting and vestibular reflexes. Cochlear damage (guinea pigs): Temporal bone of killed treated animals is removed. Inner ear is dissected under binocular to expose cochlea, and portions of organ of Corti are removed and after fixation examined by phase contrast microscopy.

Musculoirritant effects of drugs

Suggested procedures
A. Single-dose intramuscular irritation in the rabbit

Species:	New Zealand white rabbit.
Drug concentration:	50 mg in 1 ml of isotonic saline.
Treatment:	Injection with a 23 gauge needle in the mid-lumbar muscles. Injection placed from 15-20 mm deep and about the same distance lateral from the mid-line.
Observation period:	1, 3, and 7 days postinjection.
Number of animals:	2 or 3 rabbits are assigned to each observation period interval in the testing of a single compound.
Controls:	A comparable number of controls should be treated with equivalent volume of vehicle. Clinical formulation should be tested, if available.
Method:	Finally, each rabbit is electrocuted for 1 minute and the lumbar muscles perfused, then removed into fixative and later transversely sliced.
Evaluation of results:	Lesion is graded according to its 3-dimensional size, degree of hemorrhage, degeneration and necrosis using a point system to obtain numerical index of severity.

USA

B. Multiple-dose intramuscular study in the dog

Number of animals: Mostly 3 treated groups of 4 dogs each.

Controls: Control group of 4 dogs.

Treatment: Drug formulation should be same as used in man. Injection volume should be kept small, no greater than 1.5 ml, either by adjusting drug concentration or by dividing daily dose among several sites in the muscle masses. Alternating the use of bilateral injection sites from one day to the next may be useful.

Effects of drugs on the respiratory system

Species: Mice, rats, guinea pigs, rabbits, dogs and monkeys.

Exposure technique: For short term inhalation studies: preferably mask or endotracheal device. For chronic studies, usually exposure chambers.

Suggested procedures

Toxicity studies **prior to Phase I clinical trials** on inhalants intended to be administered for only a few days to any one individual.

A. Acute inhalation

Scope of study: Establishment of LC50 of test inhalant.

Species: 2 to 3, selected on the basis of pharmacological, physiological or biochemical responses.

Sex: M and F.

Exposure: Single exposure, one exposure time.

Drug concentrations: 4 or 5.

Number of animals: Sufficient numbers of each sex in each group.

Controls: For aerosolized preparations 2 control groups recommended, one treated with vehicle alone at highest concentration used for drug treated group, one unexposed group.

Duration of each exposure: From a few minutes to several hours, depending on proposed clinical use.

Variables: Deaths occurring during and after exposure.
During exposure time: signs of toxicity such as ocular and nasal irritation, respiratory distress and adverse physiological and pharmacological effects.
After exposure time: loss of body weight and alteration of behavioral, physiological and neurological responses.
Autopsy of animals which died during and after exposure. Survivors should be sacrificed at several designated post exposure intervals. Histopathological examination if necessary.

USA

B. Repeated inhalation

Scope of study:	Determination of total effects from repeated inhalation of test inhalant under normal and exaggerated use conditons.
Species:	2, one non-rodent.
Sex:	M and F.
Exposure:	Daily exposure for up to 14 exposure days, 1 to 3 different exposure durations, exposure to test and control atmospheres.
Drug concentrations:	2 to 3. One should produce some toxic effects in at least one species. At least 2 concentrations at fractions of the LC50 or multiples of the poposed therapeutic concentration, usually 3 and 10 times, are tested.
Number of animals:	Sufficient numbers of each sex of each species.
Variables:	Cardiopulmonary function, clinical chemistry, hematology, histology.
Interactions:	For inhalation anesthetics, studies on interaction of anesthetic with the adjuncts may be included.

Toxicity studies **prior to Phase II clinical trials** on a limited number of patients for specific disease control of prophylaxis.

1. Inhalant intended to be administered for up to one week.

A. Acute inhalation

Same as in Phase I, A, but with 2 or 3 additional exposure periods (use and exaggerated use).

B. Repeated inhalation

Same as in Phase I, B, but with total number of exposure days increased to 30.

2. Inhalant intended to be administered for up to 1 month

A. Acute inhalation

Same as in Phase II, A.

B. Repeated inhalation

Same as in Phase I, B, but with total number of exposure days increased to 90 and additional animals of the smaller species for periodic biochemical or physiological assays at 30, 60, and 90 exposure days.

Toxicity studies to be performed **prior to Phase III clinical trials** (large scale clinical trial of the drug).

1. Single administration clinically

A. Acute inhalation

Same as in Phase II, A.

B. Repeated inhalation

Same as in Phase II, B.

USA

2. Short term clinical use of 1 or 2 weeks duration.
   ### A. Acute inhalation
Same as in Phase II, A.
   ### B. Repeated inhalation
Same as in Phase I, B, except for the increase of the total number of exposure days to 60 days.

3. Repeated administration clinically for 4 to 12 weeks.
   ### A. Acute inhalation
Same as in Phase II, A
   ### B. Repeated inhalation
Same as in Phase II, B.

Note: During Phase III toxicity investigation, appropriate consideration should be given to metabolic, reproduction, teratogenic, mutagenic and carcinogenic potentials. These subjects are covered in the respective guidelines and the use of the inhalation route does not modify the test procedures.

USA

USA VIII: Final Report to the Commissioner, Food and Drug Administration, Agency Steering Committee on Animal Welfare Issues. U.S. Department of Health and Human Services, Public Health Service, Food and Drug Administration. August 15, 1984.

General Concept:

The FDA has no regulations requiring the use of the LD50 test. An approximation of this value is sufficient for all except a few highly toxic drugs such as some cancer chemotherapeutic agents.

The Code of Federal Regulations (21cff202) specifies information for physician labelling and prescription drugs. An overdose section includes oral LD50 values if available, but the value need not be statistically precise, and is often derived from an acute study.

This policy is confirmed in a lecture presented by Vera C. Glocklin, Ph.D., Office of Drug Research and Review of the FDA, presented at the FDA Acute Studies Workshop, Washington, D.C., November 9, 1983. The pertinent paragraph reads as follows. «It should be emphasized that there is **no** regulatory requirement for statistically precise LD50 as part of this acute toxicity characterization. An approximation of this value will generally suffice for all except a few highly toxic drugs with such narrow margins of safety that LD50 precision would be needed to determine its separability from the median effective dose.»

Further confirmation of this attitude is contained in a report on the Acute Studies Workshop sponsored by the U.S. Food and Drug Administration, November 9, 1983, prepared by the office of Science coordination, U.S. Food and Drug Administration, Department of Health and Human Services.

The following conclusions were reached:
«Although FDA requires acute toxicity data, it has no regulations requiring use of the LD50 test to assess the safety of the products it regulates.

Related to the issue of the type of data needed, there was general agreement among government and industry program representatives that the LD50 test was often credited with greater quantitative and scientific accuracy than it merits and that there are other determinants of acute toxicity such as site and mechanism of action, early or delayed lethality and recovery rate, that are better indices of toxicity and hazard than LD50 values per se.

Industry and government agencies support the development and validation of alternative methods – those using as few animals as possible and those that use no animals. However, until valid substitutes are available, animals must continue to be used to develop data to meet the responsibilities that government and industry have to protect the more than 200 million people in the U.S..»

Zimbabwe

Document reviewed:

ZIMBABWE: IFPMA Registration Compendium, compiled in March 1987 (obtained from D. Galletis, Registrar of the Drugs Control Council, on November 26, 1987).

Address of Regulatory Agency:

Drugs Control Council, P.O. Box UA 559, Union Avenue, Harare, Zimbabwe.

Note:

The above document contains a summary of the procedure for registering drugs. Marketing authorization depends on proof of safety, quality and therapeutic efficacy.

Information is required on whether or not product is registered in country of origin.

Toxicology studies:

Conditions and guidelines for the conduct of scientific studies are presently being drawn up on the lines of Nordic Council Guidelines.

Further information

on requirements for the contents of applications is contained in the Drug Control Council: «Drug Registration and Control in Zimbabwe», (Reference: B/279/35/1/85) of January 7, 1985, and «To all Applicants of Veterinary and Human Drugs» (Reference: B/279/35/3/86) of June 25, 1986.

No detailed requirements for toxicity testing are included in these documents.

Toxicological Requirements of Biotechnology Products

General concepts

The rapid developments in the area of recombinant DNA technology and production of monoclonal antibodies, and the serious and unexpected adverse effects observed with some of these substances (interferons, interleukins, etc.) have led to an intensive discussion of possible safety studies of these agents. It is recognized that biotechnology products have many special features that preclude the use of drug safety tests developed for small molecules. On the other hand, scientifically validated testing concepts have not yet been developed. The current thinking of experts from governments, industry and universities is described in several papers assembled in the book «Preclinical Safety of Biotechnology Products», Charles E. Graham, Ed., Alan R. Liss Inc., New York, 1987.

Several drug regulatory agencies have issued proposals and tentative guidelines. They are listed below with brief summaries of the contents.

USA Food and Drug Administration

1. **Document reviewed:** Points to consider in the production and testing of new drugs and biologicals produced by recombinant DNA technology. Draft November 7, 1983, Office of Biologics Research and Review. National Center for Drugs and Biologics.

> Regulatory concepts: New licence application or new drug application required for products made by recombinant DNA technology, even if product is identical in molecular and chemical structure to naturally occurring substances or previously approved product manufactured by conventional methods.
>
> Expression systems: Exact description of the technology used to obtain recombinant DNA product required.
>
> Master cell bank: Exact rules for the monitoring of quality and identity of host cells are provided. Host cells to be analyzed for reverse transcriptase and virus-like structures.
>
> Production: Detailed description of production methods. Penicillin and other beta-lactam containing antibiotics should be avoided.
>
> Purification: Exact description of method of purification. Undesirable antigenic materials, viruses, microbial contaminants and nucleic acids must be eliminated. Quality assurance procedures must be described.
>
> Physico-chemical characterization of product: Various procedures are proposed depending on the nature of the product: Amino acid analysis, partial sequence analysis, peptide mapping, polyacrylamide gel electrophoresis and isoelectric focusing, high performance liquid chromatography, circular dichroism and optical rotatory dispersion.
>
> Biological tests for identity and potency and tests for contaminants (pyrogens, viral contamination, nucleic acid contamination, antigen contamination, microbial contamination).

Toxicity tests in animals: Recombinant DNA product identical to natural substance for which pharmacology and toxicology data are available require limited toxicology. Natural compounds with minor modification require more testing. Compounds radically altered from natural substances require more extensive animal tests including carcinogenicity, teratogenicity and effects on fertility.

The specific tests which might be appropriate are best addressed on a case by case basis with the appropriate Office

2. **Document reviewed:** Interferon (IFN) test procedures: Points to consider in the production and testing of interferon intended for investigational use in humans, Office of Biologics, National Center for Drugs and Biologics. Draft (not dated).

Manufacturing process: The cell substrate for IFN production must be clearly identified, and the procedures used to obtain recombinant DNA derived products should also be described.

Inducers and purification: A clear description of biological or chemical inducers used should be provided and the adverse properties of these inducers such as toxicity, carcinogenicity, pyrogenicity should be evaluated. Removal methods and assay for residues of inducers should be provided, and specifications for inducer residues in final products should be proposed.

Purification: Same concept as described above should be employed.

Consistency of manufacture: Tests to assure consistency of the product should be described.

Final product tests including a test for pyrogenicity and extraneous toxic contaminant content.

Toxicological testing: This document does not contain any proposals for toxicity tests.

3. **Document reviewed:** Points to consider in the characterization of cell lines used to produce biological products, John C. Petricciani, M.D. Food and Drug Administration, Bethesda, June 1, 1984.

This document contains proposals for the characterization of cell lines used in biological products development, e.g. identification of cell line, presence of mycoplasms, bacteria, fungi and viruses.

4. **Document reviewed:** Points to consider in the manufacture of monoclonal antibody products for human use. Office of Biologics, National center for Drugs and Biologics, FDA. Draft (not dated).

This document discusses the production and safety of hybridoma-derived monoclonal antibody products for human use. It describes the requirements for the exact characterization of the cell system used to produce monoclonal antibodies, the production procedures, the assessment of possible viral and nucleic acid contamination and purification of the products.

Preclinical animal testing:
General concepts: Traditional toxicological test procedures are unlikely to provide information which will be relevant to use of most monoclonal

antibody products. Nevertheless, it is recommended to conduct some animal tests. It is recognized that such tests cannot detect anaphylaxis and other allergic reactions that may occur in humans.

Recommended procedures: Safety studies should be performed with limited number of animals in at least one species other than mice. Use of additional species encouraged.

Administration procedures should be appropriate to conditions of proposed clinical testing (same route, same freqency as proposed in humans). If a coupled product is used, then the actual coupled compound should be tested.

Variables: Acute toxicity, general behavior, body weight, condition at injection site, target organ histology, hematology, blood chemistry, urine analysis, tests for renal- and hepatotoxicity.

Immunopharmacological studies, e.g. half-life studies, binding studies, metabolism, clearance, biodistribution, target antigen modulation and in vivo cross reactivity whenever possible.

In vitro testing for cross reactivity. Immunohistological survey of human vital organs, blood components and intended target cells or tissues using quick frozen and chemically fixed adult and, if available, fetal tissue samples. Tissues from unrelated donors should be evaluated to screen for possible variations in phenotypic expression of potentially cross-reactive tissue antigens.

In vivo testing for cross-reactivity: Whenever possible in animals or, if possible, in perfused human organs. If not possible, clinical monitoring necessary in volunteers or patients.

France

A proposal entitled « Recommandation concernant le protocole toxicologique des interférons pour l'obtention d'une autorisation de mise sur le marché» issued by the Direction de la Pharmacie et du Médicament, Paris, 12.3.1984 and 16.3.1984 is available.

Summary of the toxicological requirements.

Single dose administration: Two species, both sexes, in one species by two routes, two weeks observation.

Repeated dose administration: Two species, one rodent, one preferably subhuman primate, three months daily injections.

Local administration: (when appropriate) at least one month.

Reproductive toxicology: Segment I and II. Exceptions must be justified.

Mutagenicity: At least one in vitro and one in vivo test, preferably assessing clastogenic effects.

Caracinogenicity: Not required.

Pyrogenicity: Rabbit test.

Local tolerance: Standard procedure including histopathology.

Safety pharmacology: In vivo assay for cardiopulmonary toxicity, in vitro study using isolated guinea pig heart, neurobehavioral studies including experiments with intrathecal injections. Effects on isolated organs.

Cell culture experiments: Cytostatic, cytotoxic and other properties.

United Kingdom

Document reviewed: Considerations for the Standardization and Control of the new Generation of Biological Products. Draft (July 1984). The National Institute for Biological Standards and Control, Holy Hill Hampstead, London NW3 6RB.

These guidelines describe research and manufacturing procedures and control procedures for recombinant DNA derived products and agents obtained by hybridoma technology. The document essentially contains descriptions of good manufacturing procedures and quality control. No toxicological requirements are discussed.

Japan

Document reviewed: The original guideline for manufacture of drug products by application of recombinant DNA technology (draft) of March 30, 1984 has been replaced by «Guideline for quality assurance on drug products obtained by cell culture», (draft) March 31, 1987.

General concept of toxicological testing: «Toxicity studies on drug products obtained by cell culture should generally be performed based on views and by methods, different from those for conventional pharmaceuticals because of their unique properties. As we have limited findings and experiences in the subject area and as we expect increased diversity in types and properties of drug products obtained by cell culture and in the applicable methods to their clinical use, we believe that it is not reasonable to establish uniform standards and methods of studies at this time point. We shall, therefore, establish the general principle of conducting scientifically pertinent studies at the given time and accumulate data in order to contribute to optimum evaluation of safety of such pharmaceuticals for clinical use, and deal with the concrete tests scope for individual pharmaceuticals on a case by case basis by giving consideration to the properties of the pharmaceuticals and the applicable methods to the clinical use.»

General note: Toxicity studies should take into consideration methods of preparation, physical properties, pharmacological actions, mechanism of action, pharmacodynamics, efficacy, dosing, etc. Contaminants are important.

Animal species to be selected with proper regard to their physiological and pharmacological responses to active components.

Route and frequency of application: as similar as possible to those intended for clinical use.

Antibody production: should be considered and monitored. Test animals with lower likelihood of producing antibodies are preferred.

Special cases: Part of toxicity tests may be omitted if active ingredients obtained by cell culture are identical to those of human-derived product which results of toxicological studies are already available. However, toxicity of contaminants must be considered.

Toxicity tests: All tests referred to below should be performed, however, the unique characteristics of biotechnological products should be taken into consideration.

Acute toxicity: Always required. Number of species: two. Only one if species available which simulates response in humans.

Subacute toxicity: To be performed with all products (except vaccines, used only once or a few times).

Antibody production: If meaningful studies are prevented by antibody production the test may be shortened.

Chronic toxicity: To be performed if appropriate. Normally on compounds proposed for prolonged clinical use, products having active components radically different from those of human-derived products, and those obtained by binding toxins and radiochemicals to monoclonal antibodies. These studies may be omitted because of antibody production or other reasons. They are difficult to conduct.

Reproduction studies: To be performed when compound contains components different from those derived from humans or if drug is likely to be administered to women who are pregnant or of reproductive age. If the drug is suspected to cause abortion, tests should be performed in primates.

These studies may be omitted if reasonable justification can be given.

Mutagenicity: Normally required. Test procedures using mammalian cells are preferred. Doubtful results should be followed by in vivo tests. Not only structural aberrations but also quantitative chromosomal aberrations should be studied by in vitro tests.

Carcinogenicity: These studies should be considered mainly for compounds administered over a long period or with suspicious structure. These studies may be omitted if reasonable justification can be given.

Dependence test and local irritation test.: To be conducted when necessary, but may be eliminated for reasonable causes.

Antigenicity test: Requirement: Conducted for pharmaceuticals which are administered clinically over a long period and those containing active components having chemical structures apparently different from those derived from humans. The studies may be omitted if reasonable justification can be given. Important is the detection of trace impurities from cells, media or purification method, and substances related to active components (analogues, aggregates, degradation products, etc.). Methods with highest sensitivity should be selected; possible interaction with active components should also be considered.

Pyrogen test: Tests in rabbit or other test methods. If compound is *per se* a pyrogen, mechanism should be studied.

Immunotoxicology: Commpounds affecting the immune system should be investigated in detail. Monoclonal antibodies should be investigated for their ability to cross-react with antigens similar but different from the target antigens.

Steroidal Contraceptive Drugs

Document reviewed: Guidelines for the toxicological and clinical assessment and post-registration surveillance of steroidal contraceptive drugs. WHO Special Programme of Research, Development and Research Training in Human Reproduction, World Health Organization, 1987, Geneva 27, Switzerland (HRP/SP.REP/87.1)

Brief summary: This document reviews the history of toxicological testing of contraceptive steroids in animals and in other non-human systems. It summarizes the requirements in various countries and discusses the success and failures of the conventional testing approach.

New concepts for toxicological testing of contraceptive steroids are developed, stressing the marked species differences with regard to reproductive physiology, hormonal control of reproductive processes, hormone receptor sensitivities and pharmacokinetics of hormonal products.

The following procedures are proposed:

Initial toxicologcal studies: These should concentrate on general tolerance, pharmacokinetics and selected endocrine effects. Single dose toxicity studies should be limited to one rodent species and, whenever possible, a limit test or a determination of the approximate lethal dose should be performed. In general no determination of the LD50 is required.

Repeated dose toxicity studies should be performed in two species, selection should, if possible, be based on pharmacological considerations and pharmacokinetics of the compound. There is no merit in conducting long-term studies with contraceptive steroids in high doses. Dose selections should be based on pharmacodynamic and pharmacokinetic considerations. Duration: not more than 6 months. Longer periods only for compounds that are very slowly eliminated.

Reproduction studies: The major emphasis is placed on effects on embryonic and fetal development. Experiments should also be conducted in the last part of gestation to investigate the potential adverse effect on the development of the genital tract. Rodents are usually suitable.

Mutagenicity studies: Tests for gene mutation in microorganisms and mammalian cells with in vivo and in vitro cytogenetic tests for chromosome aberrations are recommended. New scientific developments in the future should be incorporated in the testing procedures.

Carcinogenicity studies: If necessary, the studies should be conducted in a rodent species. Particular consideration should be given to pharmacokinetic aspects which determine dosage regimen (if possible comparable to that proposed for man).

Consideration should also be given to the possibility of reversal of proliferative changes after withdrawal of treatment.

Sex of the laboratory animal: Usually only females. In carcinogenicity studies both sexes are recommended.

Established contraceptive steroids in new delivery systems: Major emphasis placed on local tolerance of the delivery system. No need to repeat systemic toxicity studies.

New derivatives of established contraceptive steroids, e.g. long acting esters and other derivatives: These substances must be treated as new steroids unless the pharmacological action can be shown to be due to the parent steroid. In such cases, only limited toxicity studies are necessary before proceeding to clinical trials. Before marketing, detailed toxicological studies as described for new steroids must be performed.

Testing of combinations of contraceptive steroids: The estrogen to progestogen ratio which varies widely between animals and man is critical. For toxicological studies the ratio of estrogen to progestogen must be adjusted to reflect the physiological conditions.

Timing of animal toxicology and clinical trial: For phase I and IIa clinical studies: Results of single dose toxicity and limited repeated dose studies in animals must be available. For phase IIb: Repeated dose toxicity studies (long-term toxicity tests) and reproduction studies must be completed.

Before starting large scale phase III clinical trials: Long-term carcinogenicity studies should have been initiated and information on efficacy and safety of the drug in humans must be available.

Notification and Approval Procedures for Clinical Trials

General remarks

Preclinical toxicological studies are first performed to establish the safety of a new drug for clinical trials in healthy volunteers and in patients. In several countries, the extent of such animal tests is strictly regulated. It usually depends on the phase of the proposed human studies. In general, these countries also require at least notification of the health authorities regarding the intended studies in humans, and the deposition of a dossier containing the results of pharmacological and toxicological experiments conducted so far. This documentation is reviewed by the staff of the regulatory agency or an advisory board, and clinical trials can proceed after a more or less formalized approval has been issued. In other countries, the conduct of clinical trials is the responsibility of the sponsoring drug firms and the clinical investigators.

The following summary describes the notification and approval procedures for clinical trials for those countries that have, to our knowledge, issued official and written requirements or from which we have obtained authoritative personal information. Countries that are not mentioned may have an official approval policy not described in the documentation available for review.

Nordic Guidelines

Document reviewed: Drug applications. Nordic guidelines. Prepared by Nordic Council on Medicines in Cooperation with the Drug Regulatory Authorities in Denmark, Finland, Iceland, Norway and Sweden. NLN Publication No 12, Nordiska Läkemedelsnämnden. 1st edition, Uppsala November 1983.

Regulatory agencies must be notified of all clinical trials of non-registered drugs. In addition, notification of the following clinical trials is required:
- trials for new indications
- trials in patient groups not previously adequately studied
- trials with doses that are considerably higher than previously approved
- long-term trials involving large numbers of patients
- trials to determine frequency of adverse reactions
- trials involving radiopharmaceuticals

Notification must be submitted by clinical investigator. If study is conducted in cooperation with manufacturer, manufacturer or national agent must sign. If trial conducted in hospital or scientific institution the medically responsible senior physician or head of institution must also sign.

The notification is reviewed by drug regulatory agency. Administrative procedures vary from country to country.

Austria

Document reviewed: Bundesgesetz Nr. 185, über die Herstellung und das Inverkehrbringen von Arzneimitteln (Arzneimittelgesetz). March 1983.

Documentation from chemical, pharmacological and toxicological studies must be available.

For clinical trials involving the first administration of new drug to man and/or the first administration of new dosage form, an expert report by the Drug Advisory committee (Arzneimittelbeirat) must be submitted to the Ministry of Health and Environmental Protection. In addition, the clinical investigator must submit a trial protocol and notify the Ministry of the scheduled starting date of clinical trials.

Canada

Document reviewed: Health Protection Branch, Health and Welfare Canada. Guidelines for Preparing and Filing Preclinical New Drug Submissions. Drugs for Use in Humans. Draft, May 1986.

Before a clinical study may be initiated, a Preclinical New Drug Submission containing the specified information presented in a suitable form and with appropriate content must be submitted to and found acceptable by the Director. It is proposed that all submissions respecting clinical testing will be administered as follows:

Within 60 days following the acknowledgement of receipt of the Preclinical New Drug Submission, the Division charged with the responsibility for evaluation of that submission will inform the manufacturer:

1. That the submission complies or does not comply with Section C.08.005 of the Food and Drug Regulations, or
2. That the data submitted are inadequate to formulate an opinion respecting compliance and that additional data are required.

As a matter of policy, the Division will respond within 30 days of acknowledgement of receipt of preclinical submissions which are presented as protocols only (in some cases, with minimal supplementary information) and which are intended to extend, modify or further develop clinical trials for a drug which has already received a Notice of Compliance under Division 8.

In filing a Preclinical New Drug Submission the sponsor must be prepared to justify the research proposal from a scientific viewpoint and from a standpoint of ethical standards. The rights, safety and wellbeing of the research subjects must be safeguarded in accordance with the community's sense of proper conduct. The principal clinical investigator and the study sponsor have a joint responsibility for the welfare of the subject or patient. The local Independent Review Committees and the Health Protection Branch provide additional safeguards by reviewing, recommending modifications and, if necessary, disapproving the design and/or conduct of a proposed study. The Independent Review Committees should monitor all clinical studies from an ethical viewpoint and have the main responsibility for ensuring that the principles of informed consent (which in accordance with the Helsinki Declaration are a prerequisite to ethically valid research) are implemented in protecting the subjects of all proposed studies.

The Preclinical New Drug Submission should include a section on chemistry and manufacturing with information under the following headings suggested in the

«Chemistry and Manufacturing Guidelines, Preclinical New Drug Submissions 1984»: Drug substance, dosage forms, manufacturing facilities and controls.
The Drugs Directorate's «Preclinical Toxicologic Guidelines – 1981» should be consulted for the extent and type of information required for submission and evaluation by the Health Protection Branch before clinical trials are undertaken.

Chile

There are no administration rules for obtaining a licence to conduct clinical trials.

People's Republic of China

Document reviewed: Provisions for New Drug Approval. July 1, 1985.

Detailed rules on the conduct and reporting of clinical trials of new drugs are issued (Annex 6: Technical requirements for the clinical investigation of new drugs (Western drugs)) of «Provisions for New Drug Approval». No rules for notification procedures and toxicological requirements are contained in this document.

Federal Republic of German (FRG)

Document reviewed: Der Bundesminister für Jugend, Familie und Gesundheit. German Drug Law (Arzneimittelgesetz), Section 6, Protection of Humans During Clinical Trials.

Pharmacological and toxicological data must conform to current scientific standards and must be sent to the responsible federal authorities. In addition, the law defines the necessary qualifications of clinical investigators and describes informed consent procedures. No official approval is necessary.

France

The current procedure for obtaining a licence to conduct clinical trials, is:
A notification from the laboratory must be sent to the Service Central de la Pharmacie et des Médicaments before initiating clinical trials with a therapeutic objective.
Note: Clinical trials in healthy volunteers are not permitted in France.
This notification must comprise:
– The names of the analytical expert(s), pharmaco-toxicological expert(s) and of the anticipated clinical expert(s) with their professional qualifications.
– A summary of the chemical, biological, biochemical, kinetic, toxicological, galenical, analytical data, intended use, dosage, etc.
The Ministry issues a registration number which will facilitate confirmation of whether the manufacturer fulfilled the original intentions of the clinical trial, and whether the information given was valid, when the Marketing Authorization (AMM = Autorisation de Mise sur le Marché) is filed.

German Democratic Republic (GDR)

Document reviewed: Law pertaining to the drug trade (Arzneimittelgesetz) of November 27, 1986.

For each stage of clinical testing permission must be obtained from the Ministry of Health.
Domestic manufacturers submit requests to Secretariate of Control Expert Committee for the Drug Trade, Human Medicine Section (Zentraler Gutachterausschuss für Arzneimittelverkehr, Sektion Humanmedizin, ZGA).
Foreign manufacturers request permission via the advisory bureau for drugs and medical-technical products (import) of the Ministry of Health.
Test protocols and appropriate documentations must be submitted with this request. For antimicrobial drugs, a permit (Einsatzgenehmigung) from the Ministry of Health is required.
For radioactive pharmaceuticals a permit from the National Office of Radiation Safety and Radiation Protection is required.
The documentation is reviewed by 2 experts selected by the secretariats of ZGA. They must submit their opinion within 4 weeks and are present at the deliberations of the ZGA.
The approval procedure should be completed within 8 weeks.

Greece

Document reviewed: Hellenic Republic, Ministry of Health and Welfare. National Drug Organisation of Greece (E.O.F.), Ministerial Decision, December 12, 1984.

Before clinical trials may be conducted, the conclusions drawn from pharmacological and toxicological studies must be submitted to the E.O.F.. Clinical trials can only commence after permission has been granted by E.O.F.. For this purpose, an application must be submitted to the E.O.F. by the physician or dentist responsible for the trial. The application must be signed by the director of the research or clinical unit where the trial will take place.
The application must include:
– Decision of acceptance by board of directors of hospital or research establishment.
– Trial protocol.
– Detailed description of drug (chemical, pharmaceutical, toxicological, clinical).
– Adequate documentation and bibliography.
– Texts written for the information of participants and health personnel.

Hong Kong

There are no specific rules or guidelines for safety testing of new drugs and diagnostics prior to clinical investigation. However, there are legal requirements covering the use of drugs and diagnostics for clinical trials on human beings or medicinal tests on animals. Such clinical trials or medicinal tests may only be performed under the authority of a licence issued by the Pharmacy and Poisons

Board, Medical & Health Department, 1/F, Centre Point Building, 181-185, Gloucester Road, Wanchai, Hong Kong.

Hungary

Document reviewed: Prof. I. Bayer, Director-General of the National Institute of Pharmacy. Drug Registration and Drug Control in Hungary. Budapest, 1983.

Clinical trials are authorized by the National Institute of Pharmacy: the first investigators are designated by the Institute, the extension of clinical trials is granted after evaluation of the initial results by the Committee on Drug Administration and Clinical Pharmacology. The extension is to be requested by the manufacturer from the National Institute of Pharmacy: the performance of clinical trials with new, non-registered drugs is not allowed without authorization from the Institute.

Italy

Document reviewed: Ministerial Decree of July 28, 1977 (Regolamento per l'execuzione degli accertamenti della composizione e della innocuità dei prodotti farmaceutici di nova istituzione prima della sperimentazione clinica sull'uomo).

The following drugs fall under this regulation:
– Products that have never been used in man.
– New combinations of drugs already registered, or combinations of drugs already registered but in different proposed dosages.
– Drugs already registered, but proposed in different pharmaceutical formulations, containing excipients never before used, proposed for new administration routes, new clinical indications or higher dosages than previously approved.
– New pharmaceutical products already investigated or registered in other countries but declared a new drug by the Ministry of Health.
Requests for approval of clinical investigations containing details of the pharmacological and toxicological studies and the program of clinical trials must be submitted to the Ministry of Health. The application is reviewed by the «Istituto superiore di sanità» and its experts. The results of this review are communicated to the applicants.

Japan

No licence, corresponding to an IND in USA, is required to perform clinical studies. However, in accordance with Article 68 Paragraph 2 of the Enforcement Regulations, sponsors who commission clinical investigations must submit the outlines of toxicity and pharmacology tests of the investigational drug together with the clinical trial protocol to the Minister of Health and Welfare.

Luxembourg

Permission to conduct clinical trials must be obtained from the Ministry of Health.

The Netherlands

No authorization to conduct clinical trials is required. The applicant must inform the Chief Pharmaceutical officer of the proposed trial and send him documentation about the medicine and the trial.

New Zealand

Document reviewed: The Medicines Act, No. 118, Section 30, 1981.

Clinical trials of new drugs manufactured in New Zealand or imported can only proceed if appropriate scientific information is submitted to the Director General of the Department of Health and if the clinical trials and the investigators are approved on the recommendation of the Medical Research Council of New Zealand.

Singapore

Document reviewed: The Medicines (Clinical Trial) Regulations, 1978.

Clinical trials are only permitted in accordance with a certificate issued by the licencing authority. The documentation required to obtain a licence is not specified.

Spain

Document reviewed: Real Decreto 944/1978 (Sanidad y Seguridad Social). Productos farmaceuticos y preparados medicinales, ensayos clinicos.

The sponsor of the clinical trial (pharmaceutical company, clinical investigator, hospital, scientific institution) must obtain an authorization to conduct clinical trials from the Directorate of Pharmacy and Drugs. Request must be accompanied by up-to-date documentation on chemistry, pharmacology and toxicology of new drug and of clinical experience.

Sweden

In general, Sweden follows the Nordic Guidelines.
Notification of clinical trial must be in writing and sent to the National Board of Health and Welfare at least 6 weeks before intended starting date. The application is submitted to the Pharmacotherapeutic Division which reviews the data and announces its decision.

Switzerland

No notification and approval procedures for clinical trials are in force.

Thailand

Before conducting clinical trials, the investigators must submit their study protocol to «Ethical Review Subcommittee» of the Ministry of Public Health for approval. Permission from the Thai Food and Drug Administraiton for importation of drugs to be used in the trials is also required.

United Kingdom (UK)

Phase I clinical trial: Not covered by current legislation.
Phase II and subsequent clinical trials: Two notification and approval procedures are possible:
a) Clinical trial exemption (CTX). This requires submission of a summary of about 50 to 60 pages on chemical, pharmacological and toxicological data of the new drug, to be submitted according to a prescribed form. This CTX is reviewed only by the staff of the regulatory agency, and the decision is sent to the applicant within 35 days.
b) Clinical trials certificate (CTC) application. This application contains detailed information on all chemical, pharmacological and toxicological studies conducted so far. It is reviewed by the committee on Safety of Medicines (CSM) which takes up to 12 months. The decision to permit clinical trials is based on the opinion of the CSM, the same committee that will also review the documentation submitted for registration of the new drug.

United States of America (USA)

Document rewieved: Federal Register, Vol. 52, No. 53, March 19, 1987, Rules and Regulations.

Investigational New Drug Application (IND): Paragraph 312.20 Requirement for an IND.
a) A sponsor shall submit an IND to FDA if he intends to conduct a clinical investigation with an investigational new drug that is subject to paragraph 312.2(a).
b) A sponsor shall not begin a clinical investigation subject to paragraph 312.2(a) until the investigation is subject to an IND which is in effect in accordance with paragraph 312.40.
An IND may be submitted for one or more phases of an investigation:
Phase 1 includes the initial introduction of an investigational new drug into humans. These studies are designed to determine the metabolism and pharmacological actions of the drug in humans, the side effects and, if possible, to gain early evidence of effectiveness.
Phase 2 includes the controlled clinical studies conducted to evaluate the effectiveness of the drug for a particular indication in patients with desease or condition under study and to determine the common short-term side effects and risks associated with the drug.
Phase 3 studies are expanded controlled and uncontrolled trials. They are performed after preliminary evidence suggesting effectiveness of the drug has been obtained, and are intended to gather the additional information about effectiveness and safety that is needed to evaluate the overall benefit-risk relationship of the drug and to provide an adequate basis for physician labeling.

FDA's primary objectives in reviewing an IND are, in all phases of the investigation, to assure the safety and rights of subjects, and, in Phase 2 and 3, to help assure that the quality of the scientific evaluation of drugs is adequate to permit an evaluation of the drug's effectiveness and safety.

A sponsor who intends to conduct a clinical investigation shall submit an «Investigational New Drug Application» (IND), including pharmacology and toxicology information:

Pharmacology: A section describing the pharmacological effects and mechanisms of action of the drug in animals, and information on the absorption, distribution, metabolism and excretion of the drug, if known.

Toxicology: A summary of the toxicological effects of the drug in animals and in vitro.

Index

abstinence syndrome 74
abuse 122
additives 166
aerosols 43, 97, 178
allergen preparations 79
allergy 58, 68, 174, 185
anaesthetics 16, 43, 44, 56, 64, 97, 179
anemia 25, 111, 137
antibody 11, 54, 114, 174, 183, 186
antibiotics 10, 37 171, 176, 183
antidote 68
antigen 115, 183, 185
antigenic materials 183
antigenicity test 114, 187
antimicrobial drugs 193
antipsoriatics 166
artificial blood products 44
audiometry 176
Australia 38, 154
Austria 45, 190

Belgium 48
Benin 49
binding studies 185
biovailability 10, 76, 129
biodistribution 185
biological products 164
biotechnology 10, 11, 113, 183, 187
Brasil 50

Canada 52, 154, 191
cephalosporins 37
Chile 66, 192
China 67, 192

coagulation 15, 169
colorants 173
contraceptives 10, 122, 168, 188
Costa Rica 76
Cyprus 78

Denmark 79
dependence 74, 114, 123, 130
diacnostics 66, 78, 90, 146, 151, 193

EEC 20, 48, 79, 81, 85, 89
Egypt 80
electrocardiogram (ECG) 24, 34, 50, 68
electron microscopy 54, 176
electronystagmography 176
electroretinography 175

Finland 84
foreign protein test 68
France 49, 85, 192
FRG 49, 81, 192

geriatric products 119
GRD 88, 193
Greece 89, 193

hallucinogens 123
Hong Kong 90, 193
Hungary 91, 194

Iceland 93
immunosupressant agents 166

India 94
interferon 183, 184
interleukin 183
Italy 98, 194

Japan 101, 194

Kuwait 116

Luxembourg 118, 194

Malaysia 119

nephrotoxicity 37, 53, 176
Netherlands 124, 195
New Zealand 125, 195
Nordic Guidelines 33, 79, 84, 93, 127, 147, 182, 190
Norway 127
nystagmus 176

ototoxic drugs 176
overdose 10, 68, 145, 157, 181
ovulation 91

Philippines 128
photosensitization 173
phototoxicity 43, 58, 174
Poland 129
Portugal 131
propellant 159
prophylaxis 179

radioactive drugs 47, 60, 187, 190, 193
radioactivity 47
radiochemicals 187

Singapore 132, 195
South Korea 133
Spain 143, 195
sperms 42, 57, 68
Suriname 146
Sri Lanka 144
Sweden 80, 147, 195
Switzerland 49, 80, 148, 195

Taiwa 150
Thailand 151, 195
Tobago 154
tonometry 175
Trinidad 152
Turkey 155

U.K. 154, 157, 196
U.S.A. 80, 154, 196

vaccines 114, 164, 187

withdrawal 173, 189

Zimbabwe 182